SEXUALLY TRANSMITT
AND CONTRACEPꞮꞮUN

Sexual Health Promotion and Service Delivery:
Proceedings of a Consensus Workshop

Sexually Transmitted Diseases and Contraception

Sexual Health Promotion and Service Delivery: Proceedings of a Consensus Workshop

Edited by

ALI KUBBA
SARAH RANDALL

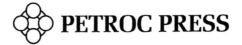 PETROC PRESS

Petroc Press, an imprint of LibraPharm Limited

Distributors

Plymbridge Distributors Limited, Plymbridge House, Estover Road, Plymouth PL6 7PZ, UK

Copyright

Published 1998 by Petroc Press, 3 Thames Court, High Street, Goring-on-Thames, Reading, Berkshire RG8 9AR, UK

A catalogue record for this book is available from the British Library

ISBN 1 900603 16 0

Typeset by Richard Powell Editorial and Production Services, Basingstoke, Hampshire RG22 4TX

Printed and bound in the United Kingdom by print in black, Midsomer Enterprise Park, Wheelers Hill, Midsomer Norton, BATH, Wilts BA3 2BB

Contents

Prologue   Ali Kubba   *ix*

Section 1   Expert Presentations

1   *Genitourinary Medicine*   R. N. Thin   3
    Current Position   3
        Management of Sexually Transmitted Diseases   3
        Cervical Cytology and Colposcopy   4
        Human Immunodeficiency Virus Infection   5
        The Health of the Nation   6
        Outreach and Community-based Services   7
    The Future   7
        The GUM–FP Interface   7
    Conclusion   9
    References   9

2   *Sexual Health of the Nation. The Case for a*
    Co-ordinated Sexual Health Service in Family Planning
    and GUM Clinics   Yvonne Stedman   11
    References   14

3   *Sexual Health: The View from General Practice*
        Colin W. Mathews   15
    Setting the Scene   15
        Basic Facts   15
        Payment of GPs   18
        Education and Training of GPs   18
    What is Already Provided?   19

Services for Women   19
Family Planning Provision   19
Cervical Screening   19
Gynaecology and Sexual Health Management   19
STD Screening   20
Male Services   21
Gaps in the Service   21
Conclusion   22

4 *Sexual Health: The Role of Commissioners*
    Rochelle Bloch   23
Introduction   23
Population Characteristics   23
Current Service Provision   25
The Purchasing Process   27
Developing a Sexual Health Commissioning Strategy   29
References   32

5 *Sexual Health – A Purchaser's Perspective of an*
    Integrated Service   Patrick R. F. Morgan   33
Introduction   33
References   45

6 *Sexual Health Promotion in Genitourinary Medicine*
    Clinics – Perspective of Patients   Jayshree Pillaye 47
Introduction   47
Patient Survey   48
Results   49
    Gender Breakdown   49
    Posters   50
    Leaflets   50
    Discussion on Safer Sex   51
    Situational Factors Leading to Unsafe Sex   51
    Contraception   52
    Prophylaxis   52
    Emergency Contraception   53
    Cervical Smears   53
    General Comments   54
    Safer Sex   54

HIV Infection   54
Perception of Visit   55
Stigma   55
Discussion   56
Summary and Conclusion   57

7 *Risk Taking and Safer Sex: Are They Irreconcilable?*
    Helen Ward   59
Introduction   59
Concepts of Risk   60
    Medical   60
    Gambling   62
    Sin and Taboo   62
Concepts of Risk – Prostitutes and their Sexual Partners   64
Prostitutes   64
Clients of Prostitutes   66
Approaches to Modifying Risk   68
References   70

Section 2   Reports from the Workgroups

8 *Workgroup 1: Components for Future Purchasing*
    Sarah Randall   73
Recommendations   73

9 *Workgroup 2: Collaboration Between Genitourinary*
   Medicine and Family Planning Services
    A. B. Alawattegama and Helen Massil   77
Introduction   77
Working Together   78
Appropriate Referral Between Services   79
Joint Protocols   80
Interface Audits   81
Conclusion   81
References   81

10 *Workgroup 3: Improving Access to Sexual Health*
    Services, and Sexual Health Promotion   83

Improving Access to Sexual Health Services   83
Service Barriers   85
People Barriers   86
Sexual Health Promotion   87

11   *Workgroup 4: Training, Evaluation and Research*
        Derek Timmins   89
     Introduction   89
     Training Needs   90
     Current Training Programmes   91
     Recommendations   91
     Subjects for Research   95
        Genitourinary Medicine   95
        Family Planning   95

Appendix 1   Consensus Workshop on Sexually Transmitted
        Diseases and Contraception: Sexual Health Promotion
        and Service Delivery   Caroline Bradbeer, Ali Kubba,
     Jayshree Pillaye, Sarah Randall and Helen Ward   97
     The Consensus Statement   97

Appendix 2   The Participants and Their Affiliations   101

Appendix 3   Acknowledgements   105

Prologue

Ali Kubba

In 1994, the Faculty of Family Planning and Reproductive Health Care (FFPRHC) of the Royal College of Obstetricians and Gynaecologists was in its second year, emerging as a lead stakeholder in the sexual health field. I had the privilege of being a Foundation Board member. I represented the Faculty on the Sexual Health and HIV Infection Working Group of the Faculty of Public Health Medicine (FPHM). I found the expertise within this group very impressive and highly complementary to the FFP's work. The idea of bringing together the various disciplines with a role in sexual health care made a lot of sense. I contacted Dr Caroline Bradbeer (my local genitourinary medicine (GUM) specialist), Dr Jayshree Pillaye (who had a sexual health remit at the Health Education Authority (HEA)), Dr Helen Ward (a public health physician with a sexual health background and training) and Dr Sarah Randall (the then Honorary Secretary of the FFP), whose organisational skills were essential for the success of the endeavour. The steering group was formed.

Invitations went to 50 participants from GUM, FP, public health, general practice, commissioners, nurses and health advisors, scientists and consumer advocates, and many others. I was pleasantly surprised by the positive response; nearly everyone invited accepted. I chose Hanbury Manor (a country retreat in Ware) as the ideal venue for the group to get to know each other and to work for over 48 hours to agree and refine a consensus.

Every participant contributed to the success of the workshop, but a few names stand out: Ms Gillian Butler opened the proceedings and made a very relevant and well-informed speech. The workgroup facilitators and rapporteurs did an excellent job in steering and then capturing the work of their groups. Peter Greenhouse provided us with the definition of sexual health that the meeting eventually adopted. David Bromham*, Roland Salmon and Mark Fitzgerald did a great deal of behind-the-scenes work to bring about a consensus and to have it eventually agreed by their organisations (FFP, FPHM and the Medical Society for the Study of Venereal Diseases (MSSVD), respectively). Dr Sheila Adams chaired the last session and was instrumental in keeping under control a bunch of excited enthusiasts!

Publishing the proceedings took longer than we wished or expected. We had to wait for the official endorsement of the consensus statement before moving forward with the publication. We then had to raise the funds required. Meanwhile several other initiatives emerged driven by the Ware momentum. The FFP and MSSVD held a successful joint conference in 1997. This is now a regular event. The Society for Advancement of Sexual Health (SASH) was established as a direct result of the Ware Workshop and should continue the work started in Ware. More importantly, several local groups and committees all over the country are applying the idea of convergence of FP and GUM and should be reaping the benefits to their service and service users.

Ali Kubba

---

*Mr David Bromham, first chairman of the FFPRHC, died in December 1996

Section 1

Expert Presentations

1 – Genitourinary Medicine

R. N. Thin

Current Position

Management of Sexually Transmitted Diseases

HISTORICAL BACKGROUND

Genitourinary medicine (GUM) has developed beyond recognition since its beginnings as venereology. The best approach to describing the position in the 1990s is to trace the evolution since the nation-wide network of clinics developed after World War I. A network of high quality clinics was established following publication of the Public Health (Venereal Diseases) Regulations (1916) which required local authorities to provide clinics for the free and confidential treatment of syphilis, gonorrhoea and chancroid[1]. These principles remain in force and were strengthened by the National Health Service (Venereal Diseases) Regulations (1974) which expanded confidentiality to include the identity of those examined or treated for any sexually transmitted disease (STD)[2]. The only exceptions were when information needed to be communicated to a medical practitioner, or a person working under the direction of a medical practitioner, and the information was for purposes of treatment or prevention. These regulations too remain in force. Both regulations are supplemented by common law confidentiality.

FACILITIES IN GUM SERVICES

In the management of STDs, staff have developed expertise in clinical diagnosis, and in the collection of samples for laboratory analysis. GUM is unique in that it supplements clinical examination with microscopy and other investigations within the clinical setting to assist in rapid accurate diagnosis. In collaboration with laboratory colleagues, systems have been evolved to ensure specimens reach laboratories in optimum condition. Laboratories supporting large clinics have a large throughput which assists in ensuring high quality. Modern computer systems facilitate rapid reporting of results and quality control. Clinics hold stocks of prepacked routine treatments; bulk purchasing and preparation reduce unit costs. Thus diagnosis and treatment of STDs in clinics is high quality and cost effective. From the outset it was recognised that there were advantages to patient care for clinics to be situated in general hospitals[1].

Partner notification or contact tracing is an essential component of STD control, and staff are trained and experienced in this vital public health measure. Much of this work is undertaken by Health Advisers who combine these skills with those of counselling[3]. It has long been recognised that the diagnosis of an STD can be a horrific experience for a patient, especially the diagnosis of genital herpes simplex which can come totally unexpectedly to patients[4], unlike the diagnosis of HIV infection for which the patient is prepared by counselling. Counselling can be very time consuming but is vital to avoid long term psychological morbidity. Partner notification and counselling offer opportunities for one-to-one health education. In addition, clinics act as a resource for other aspects of sexual health education.

Cervical Cytology and Colposcopy

When cervical screening by cytology started it was recognised that among the few health care facilities some young women accessed was a GUM clinic, so 'opportunistic' screening developed in clinics and a high proportion of abnormal smears was found, and persists, in this population[5]. This led to an increased demand for colposcopy, so clinics started to provide diagnostic, and, in some cases, therapeutic colposcopy. Medical staff with gynaecological training were recruited; this enhanced their ability to provide this service and broadened the range of expertise in the clinics.

PARTNERS IN CARE

By the 1970s GUM physicians had close links with colleagues in microbiology, virology and cytology. The main clinical liaisons were with dermatology, gynaecology and urology, while important alliances were also maintained with public health medicine. Also during the 1980s, academic departments of GUM started to develop.

Human Immunodeficiency Virus Infection

Human Immunodeficiency virus (HIV) infection and AIDS were first recognised in the UK in the early 1980s among homosexual men[6]. Many of these patients were attending, or had attended, GUM clinics and had little contact with other health care providers. It was natural for them to turn to clinics for their care and the management of their HIV disease. Since that time, much of the counselling, HIV antibody testing, and outpatient and day care for HIV-infected patients (apart from haemophiliacs) has been provided in GUM clinics. Large metropolitan clinics with big populations of HIV-infected patients have developed multi-disciplinary care involving chest medicine, dermatology, gastro-enterology, imaging, immunology, infection/infectious diseases, neurology, obstetrics and gynaecology, ophthalmology, paedi-atrics, and psychology and psychiatry. In addition, complementary medicine, dietetic, pharmacy, physiotherapy and social work services are provided. In many centres (large and small) GUM physicians are in charge of inpatients or share in their care. Centres have developed alliances with community services including primary care/general practice, community nursing, day centres, hospices, and non-governmental organisations. Some clinics developed outreach services, e.g. for HIV counselling and antibody testing.

During the 1980s there was general recognition that GUM clinics were coming under great pressure from an increasing work-load. Historically they had been under-resourced but were expected to cater for an increasing number of patients with viral

STDs, especially HIV infection. Many services were stretched to the limit of their resources. This was recognised in 1988 when a survey was carried out by the Department of Health leading to the publication of Monks *et al.*'s report which was accepted by the DOH[7]. Among the 36 recommendations was that resources should be increased for GUM and management of HIV infection. Subsequently resources were made available. A second survey was followed by advice on clinic premises[8,9].

The Health of the Nation

Before publication of the then Government White Paper, *The Health of the Nation*[10], some clinics were expanding into what has since become called *sexual health*. In addition to cervical cytology and colposcopy, they provided screening for infection in relation to termination of pregnancy, free condoms and other forms of contraception, and advice including emergency contraception, psychosexual counselling and links with pregnancy advisory services[11]. These developments have been stimulated by *The Health of the Nation*[10], and in particular there has been greater emphasis on health promotion.

The aim of the GUM clinic service is to provide free, con-fidential, easily accessible, high quality, patient sensitive, cost effective care for the diagnosis and management of STDs including HIV infection, and all aspects of sexual health including health promotion[12]. The concept is one of a seamless sexual health service. A previous recommendation was that there should be GUM and HIV infection provision in every health district[7]. With the amalgamation of health districts, this standard in service provision is no longer applicable. A more recent recommendation is that the GUM clinic service should be viewed as a national resource and that there should be provision for GUM and HIV infection services in every town and city[13]. Purchasers and providers should contract to ensure that all members of the public have ready access to these services, and should be aware that many patients with sexual health problems either do not have a general practitioner or do not wish to consult their general practitioner for these problems.

Outreach and Community-based Services

The aim of providing choice and readily available services close to where the public wishes to access them is sensible, provided high quality is maintained and confidentiality can be ensured for everyone seeking care for possible STDs. High quality includes the services on the spot and the supporting services such as laboratories. To ensure quality, all these services must be under the supervision of appropriately trained and appointed consultants.

It is also important that patients should feel free to consult their GP for sexual advice. There is greater difficulty for general practice to maintain the degree of confidentiality required for STDs. Many practitioners are happy to provide some sexual health services. However, many others feel under great pressure from recent changes in primary care[14] so are anxious to continue to refer patients (Hiscock, personal communication, 1995). The concept of total general practice fundholding raises many questions which have not yet been answered.

It is crucial that provision of community based services for a few clients is not at the expense of the main services for the majority.

The Future

Many clinics started initiatives before and after publication of *The Health of the Nation*[10]. These include the package of sexual health services already mentioned. In addition, clinics for vulval disorders have been started, staffed by consultants in GUM, gynaecology and dermatology, clinics for prostatitis with GUM physicians and urologists in attendance, and well person clinics providing general health advice. The rationale for the last mentioned is that some patients attending GUM clinics suffer from low self-esteem (Gupta, personal communication, 1995).

The GUM–FP Interface

Closer alliances are needed between family planning and well-women clinics, and GUM services. GUM physicians are concerned that family planning clinic staff screen for *Chlamydia* in isolation; GUM clinic patient populations frequently have other infections at the same time as *Chlamydia*. For example, a recent review in this department showed another infection at the same time as *Chlamydia* in 15 of 25 cases in women. Another condition that family planning clinics may investigate is vaginal candidosis. The same survey in this department showed at least one other infection with candidosis in 66 of 133 patients (Olugbile, unpublished observations, 1995). It is unclear how often multiple infections occur in family planning clinic clients. When *Chlamydia* is discovered in a woman attending a family planning clinic she is referred to a GUM clinic for further assessment, treatment, partner notification and follow-up. GUM physicians entirely agree with this principle of referral, but, how many of these women actually attend?

The healthy alliances for the screening of women before termination or the insertion of an intrauterine contraceptive device are also important initiatives which should be more widespread.

It is a requirement that trainees in GUM undergo family planning training. Thereafter the amount of family planning clinical practice varies. Some interchange of medical, nursing and, probably, health adviser staff, will ensure that both groups of professionals remain up to date concerning advances in both disciplines and maintain healthy alliances.

As already indicated, community based clinics have advantages and disadvantages. In some areas, interest has been expressed in community clinics for subgroups of the population[15] such as, for example, female teenagers. Such provision is likely to require relatively large resources. Further, what happens to male partners, and where do the clients go when they grow older? There is a requirement to notify numbers of cases of different STDs (on DOH Form KC60). How easily could this be undertaken? How well would confidentiality be maintained? Sexual health services might well do better to make their main clinics attractive and accessible to all sections of potential clients. There will be advantages in developing seamless services as outlined which will require closer alliances between GUM, family planning and related services. There may be advantages in exchanging guidelines and perhaps developing shared care guidance[16]. These will also be cost effective, appeal to purchasers, and allow the easier monitoring of quality.

Conclusion

GUM will continue to expand into sexual health. Close liaison should develop and continue between GUM and other sexual health providers including family planning specialists and general practitioners. Exchange of staff, combined meetings and shared protocols will improve and maintain quality. Services should be allowed to evolve, different arrangements will suit different situations, and no model should be imposed. There are advantages in concentrating components together to provide easy access to a confidential, high quality, cost effective, seamless service.

References

1. Public Health (Venereal Diseases) Regulations (1916). Office of the Local Government Board.
2. National Health Service (Venereal Diseases) Regulations (1974). HMSO.
3. Thin, R. N. T. (1984). Health advisers (contact tracers) in sexually transmitted diseases. *BJVD*, **60**, 269–272.
4. Carney, O., Ross, E., Bunker, C., Illos, G. and Mindel, A. (1994). A prospective study of the psychological impact on patients with a first episode of genital herpes. *Genitourin. Med.*, **70**, 40–45.
5. Young, S. M. and Malet, R. M. (1993). A study comparing cervical cytology results from a genitourinary medicine department with those of two other local populations. *Int. J. STD AIDS*, **4**, 297–299.
6. Anon (1981). Immunocompromised homosexuals. *Lancet*, **ii**, 1325–1326.
7. Monks, A., Thin, N., Trotter, S. and Pryce, D. (1988). Report of the working party to examine workloads in genito urinary medicine clinics. Department of Health, London.
8. Health Building Note 12, Supplement 1: Genitourinary medicine clinics, London, 1989.
9. Thin, R. N. T. and Lamb, J. (1990). Guidance for the planning and design of genitourinary medicine clinics. *Genitourin. Med.*, **66**, 393–398.
10. *The Health of the Nation: A Strategy for Health in England.* HMSO, London, 1992.
11. Thin, R. N. (1995). Aims and organisation of GUM/HIV infection clinic services in the UK. Abstract No 1. Joint MSSVD/NSDV Conference,

Amsterdam, 1995.

12. Association for GU Medicine 1995.

13. Association for GU Medicine 1994.

14. Anon. (1995). Tackling the GP recruitment crises. *BMA News Rev.*, Feb 22, 22–23.

15. Stirland, A. (1995). Family planning up a gum tree – the integration of family planning and genitourinary services in Australia and New Zealand. *BJFP*, **20**, 132–136.

16. Stedman, Y. and Elstein, M. (1995). Rethinking sexual health clinics. *BMJ*, **310**, 342–343.

2 – Sexual Health of the Nation. The Case for a Co-ordinated Sexual Health Service in Family Planning and GUM Clinics

Yvonne Stedman

In the UK, provision of sexual health care within family planning clinics, general practice, genitourinary medicine and gynaecology has frequently been fragmented, often isolated and sometimes incomplete. The cause of this fragmentation is that this area of sexual health care is substantial and problems within this field may be numerous and diverse, ranging from contraception, sexually transmitted infections, fertility and termination of pregnancy through to the menopausal and psychosexual. Consequently men and women will present to many different specialities according to their problem; for example, to the general practitioner or family planning clinic for contraception, the gynaecologist for infertility or genitourinary physicians for genital infections. The woman presenting to her family planning doctor or general practitioner with a vaginal discharge may well be screened for vaginal infections but not always for endocervical infections[1]. If a sexually transmitted infection, such as genital warts, is detected, and treatment given, there may be no facilities to screen for other sexually transmitted infections and it is less likely that a family planning clinic or general practitioner would have the resources to undertake contact tracing.

Two specialities to which patients with sexual health problems

11

may present are those of family planning and genitourinary medicine. Historically, family planning and genitourinary medicine services were developed separately and have continued to evolve independently of each other. Consequently, services that provide different aspects of sexual health care are staffed by nursing and medical professionals who possess specific, but different, skills and career structures. This evolution in service provision has led to a situation where men and women may receive from both services investigation and treatment of varying standards and which at times is incomplete. There is therefore a clear need for a comprehensive service for sexual health. Patients with a sexual health problem need non-judgmental and sensitive management as their care will involve not only the correct management of their presenting problem but may also involve discussion of their sexual history with follow up of their partner(s). This should be an integral component of all sexual health care provision.

The specialities of family planning and genitourinary medicine are both concerned with preventing adverse consequences of sexual activity, specifically, unintended pregnancies and genital infections. Unfortunately, the most effective methods of contraception offer little, if any, protection against sexually transmitted diseases and some contraceptive methods may even increase the risk that a sexually transmitted disease will be acquired from an infected partner. Conversely, the contraceptive methods that are most effective at preventing the spread of sexually transmitted diseases are less effective as contraceptives[2,3]. Until recently the emphasis in family planning clinics had been on the provision of a service which would enable men and women to prevent and/or to plan pregnancies, with the problem of genital infections being regarded as a secondary consideration. The converse is the situation in genitourinary medicine clinics where the emphasis has been on diagnosing and treating sexually transmitted diseases in both patient and partner(s) with contraception being a consideration only in regard to the prevention of sexually transmitted diseases.

More recently the emergence of HIV infection has sharply focused attention on the need for an effective contraceptive method that protects against both infection and pregnancy.

Although publicity and efforts at health education with regard to HIV have increased the public's awareness of sexually transmitted diseases and their prevention, there is concern that a shift to barrier contraception will result in usage of less reliable contraceptive methods, with obvious consequences. Promotion of the 'Double Dutch' concept[4] is the only effective technique that currently aims to protect against both pregnancy and sexually transmitted infections. It is also vital that, if a barrier method is used, men and women are made aware of emergency contraception.

FP and GUM are seeing overlapping groups of patients, and not different groups of patients. Any 'at risk' behaviour that puts patients at risk of unintended pregnancy will also put them at risk of sexually transmitted infections. Sexually transmitted infections are not problems of minority groups; everybody is at risk.

Sexually active women and men need to be given straightforward, correct, factual information about the possible risks of sexual activity and the opportunity to discuss such matters in an appropriate environment. Such a process will aid and support the evolution of rational decision making among those most at risk.

Strategies for providing an integrated sexual health service will differ depending on the characteristics of the population to be served and of the existing services. While the provision of all sexual health services under one roof may be the ideal[5] and entirely appropriate in some circumstances, it may not be so in other settings[6]. Realistically in the short term it is unlikely to prove achievable for most health authorities. Therefore, in practice, collaboration, liaison and sharing of skills of those concerned with the delivery of sexual health care may be a way of providing men and women with appropriate care and treatment. Collaboration between these two specialities is achievable without undue cost and organisational complexity by recognising the common clinical goal of meeting all the sexual health needs of service users of both disciplines. The sharing of nursing and medical staff, either on a short- or long-term basis, and combined meetings, ensure that staff share and disseminate their knowledge and training. This interchange allows the breaking down of the perceived stigma of genitourinary medicine clinics among their staff and patients alike. All family planning clinics should have facilities to enable screening for vaginal and cervical infections, and an agreed protocol regarding the referral of patients to genitourinary medicine. Feedback, including the GP when confidentiality allows, will ensure continuing and effective collaboration and liaison. Similarly, contraceptive provision should be made available to those attending genitourinary medicine departments. Patients would then attend a service in which nursing and medical staff have both knowledge of, and confidence in, both disciplines.

All doctors and nurses faced with a patient with a sexual health problem should be aware of their own limitations in knowledge, skills and investigative procedures so that patients can be appropriately referred when necessary.

A holistic approach to the provision of sexual health care for men and women, which combines care with education, and disease management with preventative interventions, is the only way to provide a rational service.

References

1. Stedman, Y., Higgins, S. and Chandiok, S. (1995). The management of genital infection in women attending family planning clinics in the north west of England. *BJFP*, **21**, 10–12.
2. Cates, W. Jr and Stone, C. (1992) Family planning – sexually transmitted diseases and contraceptive choice: a literature update. Part I. *Fam. Plann. Perspect.*, **24**, 75–84.
3. Cates, W. Jr and Stone, C. (1992). Family planning – sexually transmitted diseases and contraceptive choice: a literature update. Part II. *Fam. Plann. Perspect.*, **24**, 122–128.
4. Doppenberg, H. (1993). Contraception and sexually transmitted diseases: what can be done? Experiences and thoughts from the Netherlands. *BJFP*, **18**, 123–125.
5. Greenhouse, P. (1994). A sexual health service under one roof: setting up sexual health services for women. *J. Mat. Child Health*, **19**, 228–233.
6. Stedman, Y. and Elstein, M. (1995). Rethinking sexual health clinics. *BMJ*, **310**, 342–343.

3 – Sexual Health: The View from General Practice

Colin W. Mathews

Setting the Scene

Basic Facts

1. INDEPENDENT CONTRACTOR STATUS

This means that any change in the working practice of a GP is usually brought about following negotiation with the GMSC or by Government imposition. The GP contracts to provide agreed General Medical Services to the patients on his/her list.

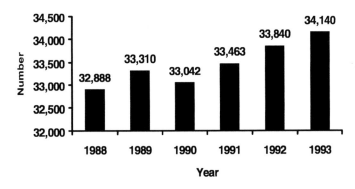

Figure 3.1 Doctors in general practice

2. MANPOWER CHANGES

Doctors have fewer patients on average today than they did 10 years ago. Practices with list sizes over 2500 have fallen from 21% in 1983 to 8% in 1993. The ratio of GPs to every 100 000 people is 54.6. There has been a significant increase in the number of GPs working in Great Britain since 1988 although these doctors may not all be full-time principals (Figure 3.1).

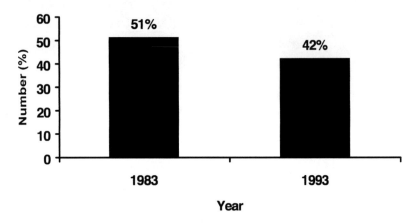

Figure 3.2   Percentages of practices with three GPs or less

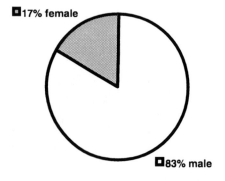

Figure 3.3   Males to females in general practice, 1983

Smaller partnerships of three doctors or less have reduced from 51% in 1983 to 42% in 1993 (Figure 3.2). So it appears that the tradition of the family doctor taking care of all aspects of a patient's health may eventually give way to the large polyclinics.

3. MALE/FEMALE RATIO

Twenty-five per cent of all GPs are female, up from 17% in 1983 (Figures 3.3 and 3.4), and 50% of trainees are female (Figure 3.5).

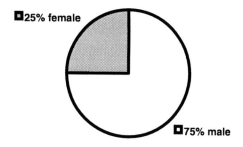

Figure 3.4   Males to females in general practice, 1993

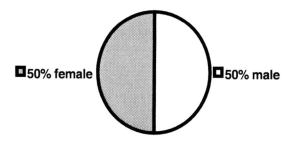

Figure 3.5   Male to female GP trainees, 1994

This increase in the number of female practitioners available has revolutionised the provision of female sexual health services, as studies have shown that female patients, on average, prefer a female practitioner for this aspect of their health.

4. FUNDHOLDERS/NON-FUNDHOLDERS

As of April 1994, there were almost 9000 GPs in over 2000 fund-holding practices, covering over one third of the population. This figure is likely to rise further in 1995 and 1996.

5. PROVISION OF SERVICES IN PRACTICE

Despite the large increase in their numbers, GPs are working harder than ever and are providing a far wider range of services. Almost without exception, all practices now provide family planning, maternity medical services and cervical cytology screening. The vast majority of GPs also offer health promotion programmes with 94% doing child health surveillance.

6. PURCHASE OF SERVICES FROM OTHER PROVIDERS

Increasingly GPs are becoming involved as fundholders, com-missioning groups or locality purchasers. In these groups they can help identify the healthcare needs of the local community and seek out providers from whom to purchase the service.

With the stronger development of the primary care team, and practice nurses playing an increasing role within practices, many GPs can expand the range of services offered to their practice population.

Payment of GPs

General practice is not a salaried service.
   Payment is made up of:

1. Practice allowance
2. Capitation fees
3. Item of service and target payments
4. Postgraduate education payments
5. Health promotion payments

As a result of capitation fees and item of service payments, GPs may earn more by having a greater number of patients and by offer-ing them more and more services. This may lead to difficulties in quality control, as has been highlighted by the recent problems in variations in cervical smear techniques between different GPs.

Education and Training of GPs

Training GPs in sexual health and FP is not compulsory. Often the only training received may be at undergraduate level. If GPs then wish to have further training in a particular field, they must still make provision for the ongoing care of their patients. At present a GP may offer family planning and cervical cytology services without proof of previous training.

What is Already Provided?

Services for Women

MATERNITY CARE AND UNPLANNED PREGNANCY COUNSELLING PROVISION

GPs, usually through a shared care system, already offer maternity care to the majority of patients. An aspect of this also involves counselling those with an unplanned pregnancy and onward referral for termination, if requested.

Family Planning Provision

With the contraction in family planning services from hospital and community clinics, more and more pressure is being put on GPs to ensure that they can meet the needs of all of their patients. GPs also counsel and arrange surgery for male patients requesting vasectomy.

Cervical Screening

With the introduction of target payments for GPs, cervical screening has seen a marked increase in the screening of eligible women (Figure 3.6). This increase in cervical cytology screening by GPs has already shown a reduction in the annual rate of deaths from cervical cancer (Figure 3.7).

Gynaecology and Sexual Health Management

As part of general medical service provision, the GP provides diagnosis and advice on management of a whole range of female problems. Hormone replacement therapy (HRT) has become increasingly used in the management of menopausal symptoms. Detection and early referral of uterine and ovarian malignancies is also an important function of the GP.

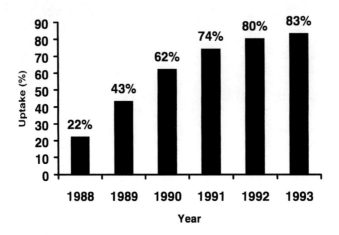

Figure 3.6   Uptake of cervical smears, age 20–64

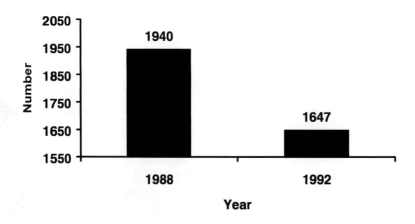

Figure 3.7   Deaths from cervical cancer

STD Screening

As GPs become more aware of the risks of chlamydial infection, more practices are able to offer a detection service. A study by

Dr Pippa Oakeshott on women attending three inner-London general practices found that screening detected 7.6% positive cases of *Chlamydia* from 1019 women[1].

A smaller survey done in my own practice in Northern Ireland shows a 7.4% positive rate with selective screening of patients. Unfortunately, many practices are still not aware of *Chlamydia* and do not have the facilities to take appropriate samples.

Male Services

As part of their provision of general medical services, GPs will provide a wide range of advice and treatment for various sexual and genital health problems. Suitable screening tests for STDs are, however, not often carried out in general practice.

Gaps in the Service

1. QUALITY OF CARE

With such a wide range of professionals providing these services, it is difficult to gain uniformity in management and it is extremely difficult to ensure that skills and knowledge are appropriately updated.

2. SERVICES FOR MEN (MANY GAPS EXIST)

- Limited condom provision in general practice.
- No item of service payment for male FP advice.
- No easy screening for GU problems.
- Young men rarely attend GPs for sexual health advice.

3. ADOLESCENT SEXUAL HEALTH

General practice is often not seen by clients as the correct setting for the provision of adolescent advice.

4. GAY MEN'S HEALTH

GP service is still seen as homophobic except in the shared care management of AIDS.

5. REGIONAL VARIATIONS IN THE SERVICE

The prevalence of GU disease varies greatly around the country and GPs might not be sufficiently motivated to provide or purchase a GUM service.

6. GENERAL PRACTICE LISTS/PARTNER NOTIFICATION

GPs provide services to a finite number of patients who are registered to that practice. Hence in the management of STDs, partner screening and treatment may not always be easy.

Conclusion

General practice has an important role to play in the development and provision of a comprehensive package of sexual health and family planning care.

It is evident that GPs have accepted cervical screening as part of their general practice provision, and hence, with extra training, GPs, especially female GPs, will be able to offer a full package of sexual health screening.

Adolescents and young men will never be adequately dealt with by traditional general practice and the provision of anonymous youth clinics will have to continue to be purchased by, or on behalf of, GPs.

The quality of expertise provided in GUM clinics for a wide range of problems cannot be matched in general practice and GPs should fight to secure locally based GUM provision.

References

1. Oakeshott, P. and Hay, P. (1995). General practice update: Chlamydia infection in women. *Br. J. Gen. Prac.*, **45**, 615–620.

4 – Sexual Health: The Role of Commissioners

Rochelle Bloch

Introduction

I am going to describe how Ealing, Hammersmith and Hounslow (EHH) Health Agency is approaching the development of a commissioning strategy for sexual health. This will include some discussion of the local epidemiology, the population characteristics, the type and range of the services that we have, and the issues that have prompted us to take this strategic direction.

Ealing, Hammersmith and Hounslow Health Agency combines both a district health authority (DHA) and a family health services agency (FHSA), and for management arrangements we were formed in 1993 after the reconfiguration of district health authorities in the North West Thames Region. However, staff were not operating from one site until 1994. We therefore spent the first year working at about four different sites over a fairly large area of west London, trying to pull together a picture of the new Authority. Within our boundaries we cover three London boroughs, three acute and four community/mental health trusts, and we have two custodial institutions (Wormwood Scrubs Prison and Feltham Young Offenders Unit), as well as Terminal 4 at Heathrow Airport (Figure 4.1).

Population Characteristics

Our population is estimated at 640000. Out of it, 11% are aged 10–14 and 5% are aged 15–19, with over 26% of the total popula-

tion coming from ethnic minority communities, mainly Asian. We
also have black African, Afro-Caribbean and Irish communities as
well as quite large refugee communities (mainly middle eastern
and Armenian). Like all health authorities covering inner city
areas, we have high levels of deprivation and homelessness, drug
abuse and HIV.

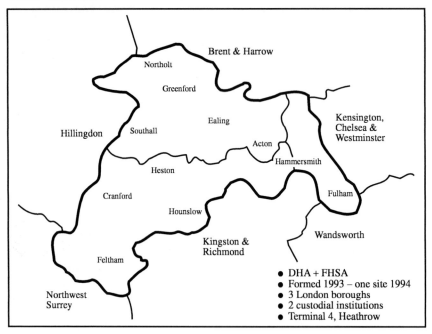

Figure 4.1   Ealing, Hammersmith and Hounslow Health Agency

With respect to sexual health, we currently have the fourth
highest prevalence of HIV and AIDS in England and Wales. To
date, there have been 710 AIDS cases reported of which 253 were
alive in March 1994. This represents 34% of the North West
Thames total[1]. In addition, we have anecdotal reports that over
1200 people are known to social services and most of those are
symptomatic.

These cases are spread differentially with about 60% in
Hammersmith and Fulham, about 25% in Ealing and about 15% in
Hounslow, with some diversity of population characteristics
between boroughs. Ealing and Hounslow tend to have a higher
than average proportion of women and children from African
communities affected, whereas Hammersmith and Fulham tend to

follow the national pattern – mainly gay men. We are also aware that in Hammersmith and Fulham it is predicted that one in a hundred men is HIV positive.

Other sexually transmitted diseases appear to be less of a problem. We have three GUM clinics – one in each borough, with a total of 35000 attendances every year. However, half of those are at one clinic where a substantial proportion of those attending are from other districts. We are in the process of recruiting a sexual health information officer to develop local surveillance systems so that we can get a much better understanding of the data and to link this in with the regional surveillance work being developed at St Mary's Hospital Medical School.

With regard to fertility, we have 170000 women aged 16–49 with a predicted 10000 births in the next year. There is a higher than average teenage pregnancy rate, particularly in Ealing, Hammersmith and Fulham, but we are also aware that the termination of pregnancy rate in Hammersmith and Fulham for the 24–34 age group is double that of the other two boroughs[2]. There is clearly work to be done to improve this situation.

Current Service Provision

The current service configuration has been inherited from a range which grew up within previous authority boundaries and did not naturally have a strategic direction. We have four acute HIV treatment centres, including two separately managed services within one trust at the moment, three GUM clinics, three maternity units, specialist fertility services at the Hammersmith Hospital, three community family planning services, and a health promotion agency which is actually located within the health agency building rather than being based in a trust.

There are 185 general practices and 365 GPs, with only 27 fund-holders. We have a very high number of single handed GPs and we have a very high priority to develop primary care. Seventy eight per cent of practices (70% of GPs) provide contraceptive services, which includes fitting IUDs.

We do have some examples of good practice in the sexual health area, some having been recently developed. There are borough-based sexual health teams co-ordinated by our health promotion unit which is based within the health agency. The teams currently operate in two boroughs and are multi-disciplinary, including GUM consultants, family planning staff and health visitors. They work together and go into schools to deliver common messages about sexual health promotion, and it seems to work well for everyone involved. We have supported curriculum development, mainly in secondary schools, although there are plans to work with primary schools, particularly to look at sexual health policies.

HIV prevention work in prison is very well developed and includes training prison officers, developing courses with the prison inmates themselves, using comic book styles and running regular health fares in one of the wings. We have also tried to develop the idea of multi-disciplinary HIV training with staff teams: family planning, maternity and primary health care, which introduced significant quality features as part of service development.

We also have a GP condom scheme. GPs cannot prescribe condoms, which has always been a problem, and EHH have invested £30 000 for the last two years in supplying condoms to GPs. GPs and practice nurses have to undergo training to get on the scheme, including developing criteria for the provision of condoms. The scheme is currently being evaluated and preliminary results show that practice staff find the supply of condoms very useful in teaching people how to use condoms, but would not envisage providing an ongoing supply. The training has been helpful for GPs in addressing a range of sexual-health-related problems.

A GP integrated-care project is operating between Hammersmith and Ealing Hospitals. This is a three-year research project funded by the region which is due to report shortly. Primarily it is investigating how to involve GPs in the care of people with HIV and AIDS, looking at what systems are appropriate and developing GP-friendly approaches.

In response to the recent unlinked anonymous HIV testing data, we have proceeded to improve our ante-natal HIV testing by having specialist midwives in two of our maternity units. We have also produced maternity services consumer information booklets, a guide for local women about what services are available and what they should expect from the services both in preconceptual care and antenatal care.

A dedicated HIV ward has opened at Ealing Hospital and is witnessing rising activity for both in-patient and day care episodes.

The Purchasing Process

One of the things people have talked about throughout this conference is how services need to be better co-ordinated. I think that there is sometimes a perception among providers that this could easily be solved if only the purchasers would decide what they want. However, as indicated in Table 4.1, the organisation of how services are purchased is no less complex than how they are provided.

Table 4.1 How services are currently purchased

HA directorate/unit	Services purchased
Acute care[1]	Maternity, gynaecology, fertility, HIV/AIDS cure, GUM, TOP
Primary care[1]	• FP/well women, health visiting, school nursing • HIV prevention (training and counselling in general practice)[2] • Pharmacy needle exchange
Community care[3]	• HIV community services (NHS, voluntary organisations, local authority) • HIV prevention (HPU, local authority, voluntary organisations, prison services) • Substance misuse services
Health gain	HPU, schools, local authority

[1]Locality purchasing
[2]Privider development unit
[3]Care group purchasing

Notes: 10 people commission this portfolio of services.
Total resources ≈ £30 000 000 (£10 000 000 HIV) – 5% EHH total allocation.

Currently sexual health services in EHH are purchased across four purchasing directorates, and about 10 different people commission this portfolio of services. It is worth noting that our primary care directorate covers both the GPs' contracts and contracts for the primary care services provided by our community health trusts. So family planning, all aspects of it, is purchased within one directorate, which is good news.

The primary care provider development unit provides direct training for GPs. Contracting for HIV services occurs in both acute and community care directorates. In addition, the health gain directorate, which incorporates public health, directly contracts with health promotion for sexual health promotion services in addition to those purchased within the HIV prevention contract.

It is currently estimated that £18 000 000 is invested in this portfolio (£10 000 000 of which is HIV money) and this represents 5% of the health agency's total budget. This is clearly a substantial amount of money and one might wonder why we have made so little progress in strategically reviewing these services. The reason is easier to understand if you consider that as purchasers we spend 60% of our time on contract monitoring. This has entailed disaggregating funds, especially managing the shifts that arose out of the reconfiguration of health authority boundaries and having to split trust contracts between two major purchasers. Also we have to set baseline activity; three of our trusts are new and had not really done much of this work before. We have also started to develop some quality standards that we can actually measure. All this work clearly has to develop collaboratively with trusts and is ongoing.

A further 30% of my time is spent on community care, involving joint planning and commissioning forums with three local authorities. This is very time consuming and involves developing criteria for joint funding of residential placements for palliative and respite care for HIV, and, until recently, also working on residential placements for drug users.

I would therefore estimate that only about 10% of the time is actually spent on service development and the whole area of needs assessment and strategic planning. Again this cannot just be internal and means working with each of our boroughs. In addition, EHH works with other London-based HIV purchasers to try to develop a strategic approach, especially around maintaining the stability of the voluntary sector, which is actually quite large in the HIV community.

We have completed some service reviews. A recent review of the termination of pregnancy service resulted in a tender and the establishment of a central booking service feeding into five providers. We had a review of GUM services which ended up with revised quality standards after extensive site visits. A family planning service review is now in its second draft and one of the outcomes is that there is going to be a more in-depth audit of the services in the Hammersmith and Fulham area. Another recommendation was to try to access young people's views in a variety of local settings and not just in clinics, and to identify what they really want from family planning services.

Developing a Sexual Health Commissioning Strategy

The prompt for developing a sexual health strategy has been that several common themes emerged from all these reviews. The key issues are:

- Uptake of services by hard-to-reach populations and at-risk groups including ethnic communities, young people including young gay men, drug users, homeless people and the refugee communities. There was a need to look at all these services with respect to opening hours, provision of interpreting services and improving publicity.
- The effect of open access services and the confidentiality inherent in the venereal disease legislation on how well we can obtain a good picture of the local epidemiology of STDs. There is a need to obtain much more robust data on sexual health in EHH.
- The need to develop and encourage clinical audit on a multi-disciplinary basis and develop joint audit between GPs and community family planning services.
- The need to review the extent of collaboration and integration

between services, what it means in practice and what it looks like in contracting terms.

- To improve the quality and consistency of client information, to ensure that all practitioners are giving out the same messages.
- Look at the role of health advisors and other specialist posts in sexual health, and improve consistency and parity between job descriptions in each trust.
- Extend team training to cover all aspects of sexual health rather than simple HIV awareness, and respond to concerns of reception staff about how to deal with difficult, angry or distressed clients.
- The need for outreach work to be better co-ordinated and targeted to populations with greatest need. We must identify measurable outcomes, be they clinical or press related.
- A need to review client confidentiality and make sure the same standards apply across all the services. We need to be able to access service user views and to make sure we're doing it right.

The health agency therefore decided to develop a strategic commissioning framework for all sexual health services. There are obviously a number of constraints and external factors which will circumscribe this process. In financial terms, EHH is going to be a heavy capitation loser and therefore any changes have to be in terms of resource shifts rather than new money. The policy context has been set out in *The Health of the Nation* and guidance on community care means we have to make sure to address the local priorities for each borough. In addition there are the operational constraints of the commissioning process, which require the production of annual purchasing plans and compliance with financial standing orders, which mean that we need to tender for any new services or changes over a certain amount of money. It is likely that any change is going to take quite a long time to implement, which is probably a good thing.

The aims and objections of the strategy are shown in Table 4.2. The terms of reference and a three-year investment plan are detailed in Table 4.3.

Table 4.2   Aims and objectives of the sexual health commissioning strategy

To define the most appropriate pattern of services required to improve the sexual health of the resident and catchment populations of EHH and to identify the purchasing shifts necessary to achieve it.

Objectives:

- To reduce the incidences of STDs
- To reduce the number of unwanted pregnancies and consequent terminations
- To ensure high quality, accessibility and acceptability of service provision
- To ensure value for money

Table 4.3   Terms of reference and three-year investment plan

- Agree a definition of 'sexual health'
- Identify component service elements
- Review level and appropriateness of current provision
- Identify changes in provision to reduce gaps, duplication and overlap
- Agree quality standards and outcomes
- Develop a three-year investment plan to achieve the necessary resource shifts
- Consult widely on recommendations

It will be important to consult widely at each stage. It is not planned to have providers as part of the strategy steering group but they will be involved throughout the process and any interim papers that are produced will be circulated widely for consultation.

Service areas that may need to be included in this strategy are wider than just family planning and GUM. As purchasers we need to embrace the best of what are traditional sexual health services, to make sure that the practice and messages are consistent and that mechanisms for interlinking and referring between services are actually working on the ground.

References

1. *AIDS/HIV Quarterly Surveillance Tables*, PHLS CDSC, December, 1993.
2. OPCS, 1992.

5 – Sexual Health – A Purchaser's Perspective of an Integrated Service

Patrick R. F. Morgan

Introduction

Many purchasing organisations are presently in the process of merging both as health authorities and with FHSAs. These changes will lead to a number of opportunities and it is important that providers understand the needs of purchasers in order to work together with them to provide the structures and services that are needed for the future.

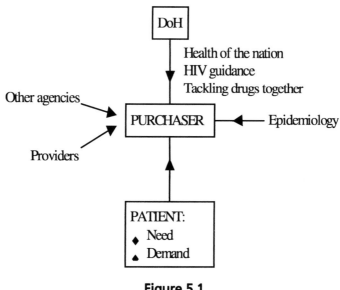

Figure 5.1

Purchasers have a number of sources of guidance from the Department of Health from which both general and earmarked funding is allocated. Included in this guidance are the requirements of *The Health of the Nation, HIV Strategies* and *Tackling Drugs Together*. It is important to remember that chief executives of commissioning authorities will be expected to account for action taken in meeting Government targets. In addition, the purchasers are balancing the epidemiological information from which needs assessments are undertaken, and which, from a public health point of view, will be community based information, along with the needs and demands of patients. In addition, the purchasers consider the services and plans for such services made by providers, and have a responsibility for co-ordinating programmes between providers and other agencies.

The Health of the Nation objectives relevant to sexual health:

- To reduce the incidence of HIV infection
- To reduce the incidence of other sexually transmitted diseases
- To reduce the incidence of invasive cancer of the cervix
- To provide effective services for diagnosis and treatment of HIV and other STDs
- To reduce the number of unwanted pregnancies – especially in the under 16's
- To ensure the provision of effective family planning services for those people who want them
- To reduce the number of women smoking at the start of their pregnancy

Ref: *The Health of the Nation*

Figure 5.2

It must be remembered that while practitioners have the technical ability to achieve many of these targets, there are huge challenges raised by the way in which services are delivered (for example, to young people). Purchasers therefore have to be informed by the findings of health systems' research in this field and look critically at whether provider management structures are able to deliver appropriate and integrated programmes that are likely to be effective. In addition, there are social, moral and religious issues that have to be considered in order to achieve these targets.

Sexual health services have a part to play in screening for cervical cancer.

Overall, the target – to reduce the incidences of gonorrhoea among men and women aged 15–64 by at least 20% by 1995 – has already been achieved. However, STDs tend to be concentrated in 'at risk' groups and overall prevalence/incidence rates may mask underlying problem areas. There are, for instance, worrying trends in *Chlamydia* rates in the Thames regions, particularly in younger people. While this data may well be influenced by a number of different variables, the graph and histograms (Figures 5.2–5.5) illustrate trends that give some cause for concern.

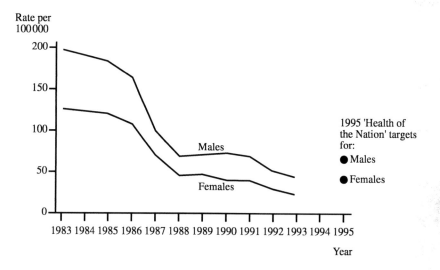

Figure 5.3   New cases of gonorrhoea in GUM clinics, England and Wales, 1983–93. (Courtesy PHLS Communicable Disease Surveillance Centre, January, 1995.)

In many rural areas, *Chlamydia* is not screened for to an extent which would allow for the calculation of proper prevalence or incidence rates. *Chlamydia* has been described as 'public health enemy number one' because of its lack of symptoms. Further population data is urgently needed to better understand the epidemiology of this infection.

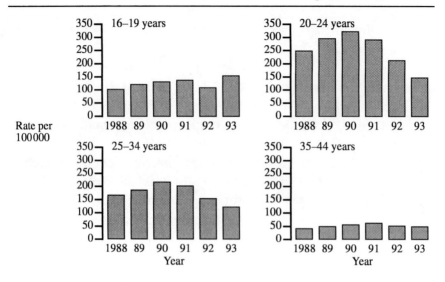

Figure 5.4   New cases of gonorrhoea in males, Thames regions, 1983–93. (Courtesy PHLS Communicable Disease Surveillance Centre, January, 1995.)

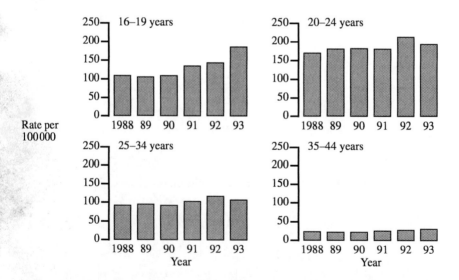

Figure 5.5   New cases of genital herpes in females, Thames regions, 1988–93. (Courtesy PHLS Communicable Disease Surveillance Centre, January, 1995.)

In most family planning clinics, attendance by under 16-year olds is increasing. However, the realisation that young peoples' risk behaviour includes not only 'sex' but also alcohol, drugs and tobacco, and that their real need for information and help encompasses many other general health issues, leads to the obvious conclusion that more integrated services in all of these fields is the natural way of realising health gains. Staff providing sexual health services should be prepared to provide counselling and advice on drug and alcohol issues and to be able to identify people with problem use so that appropriate referral to a specialist service may be made. Providers should remember that there may well be common funding sources between HIV, drug misuse, family planning and GUM services.

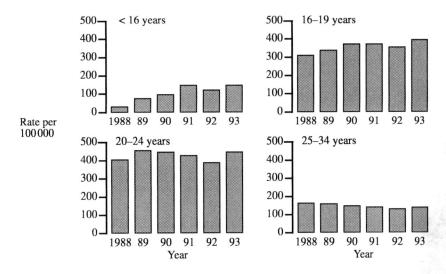

Figure 5.6 New cases of *Chlamydia* in females, Thames regions, 1988–93. (Courtesy PHLS Communicable Disease Surveillance Centre, January, 1995.)

The Health of the Nation advocates that:

'*The Government, health services, local authorities, the voluntary sector, the education sector and users of services will need to work together to meet these targets. There needs to be a willingness to address and discuss attitudes and behaviour in what are very sensitive areas.*'

It should be noted that within the green paper *Tackling Drugs Together* there is a similar requirement for health services to work with other agencies in order to deliver better care. Purchasers may well be looking for evidence of inter-agency working in provider's business plans.

> *'Sexual health, however, is not restricted to the control of disease.*
> *It also encompasses family planning and family planning services,*
> *which play an important part in the health of children and the well*
> *being of families by reducing the number of unwanted pregnancies*
> *and births.'*

(Source: *The Health of the Nation*)

It is interesting to note that *The Health of the Nation* refers to 'sexual health'. This implies a more holistic approach to a group of specialist services related to sexual function. The reality is that family planning services have, in many cases, been contracted for separately from GUM services, HIV and AIDS programmes (Figure 5.7).

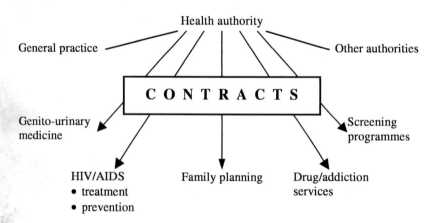

Figure 5.7

In many cases this has led to services developing independently. Generally, this group of services is a relatively small one, and in many of the more rural areas, services such as family planning are not always consultant led, nor in many cases are they part of a 'clinical' directorate. In many cases this has also led to difficulties with developing these services as they do not have a medical voice at the appropriate level in the trust. In addition, the contracting process may well bypass them and be undertaken by people who may not know the service well. In 1995 many purchasers and/or providers recognised this and are working to remedy it.

Many purchasers are concerned to bring together a range of services that, from the patients' point of view, are comprehensive, equitable and easily accessed. The Venn diagram in Figure 5.8 shows examples of the sorts of services that may well be brought together, some being in the community, some in primary care, and some in the acute sector. Some, such as health promotion, may be delivered by health authorities through public health departments. The overlap of these services is considerable and it is important therefore to be clear of the core business of each of these areas and the areas which appropriately should overlap with other programmes or be undertaken by suitably trained staff in other disciplines.

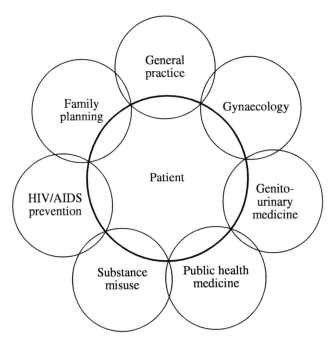

Figure 5.8   The types of services that may well be integrated

A number of services fall under the sexual health label, and may include the following:

Possible components of a sexual health service:

- Contraception
- Planning pregnancy
- Screening
- Termination of pregnancy
- Emergency contraception
- Sexually transmitted diseases
- Infertility
- Psychosexual problems
- Menopause

Within programmes there is a strong theme of prevention.

Preventing:

- Unintended pregnancy
- Genital (and other) infections
- Male and female genital carcinomas (cervix, breast, prostate, testes)
- Smoking and related diseases
- Obesity and related diseases

These services are provided by both general and specialist practitioners.

Services:

- General practitioners
- Specialist practitioners:
    Family planning and reproductive health care
    Genitourinary medicine
    Community gynaecology
- Plus
    FP nurses/practice nurses
    Health advisors

From the purchasing perspective, it is important to bring together specialties in a way which preserves their specialist functions, but at the same time builds a team of people with different skills able to support a strategy of integrated sexual health provision. The key is teamwork and recognition of the different specialist functions. Public health medicine has a key role to play in bringing together the views of different specialties. Figure 5.9 suggests a pyramid which, for the purpose of purchasing, shows public health at the top, leading in ensuring the integration of specialties. Target groups are identified and overlaps of services utilised to enhance integration.

Purchasing

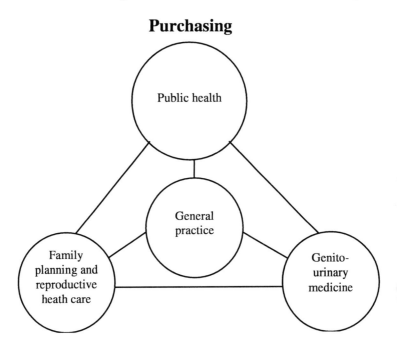

Figure 5.9   The 'purchasing' pyramid

It should be remembered that 10% of all health visiting time, even when health visitors are employed by GP fundholders, is available to health authorities for public health programmes. Clearly, sexual health programmes are an area where health visiting could be particularly effective. Examples of a potential role for health visiting is involvement in infection control for GUM, tackling teenage pregnancy for family planning and supporting cervical screening programmes in general practice.

General practice functions in both a purchaser and provider role. Total fundholding may well be seen as a potential threat both to

GUM and to family planning services if GPs decide they wish to provide these services themselves. In my view, GUM is an important component of a public health programme in that its main responsibility is to control a number of infectious diseases transmitted between humans. It should be seen as a function of similar importance to tuberculosis control. Family planning services also have an important public health function, particularly where they are undertaking targeted work which general practice either does not wish to undertake or is unable to undertake. Examples of this include targeting services to young people through outreach work. Clearly, one of the other advantages of family planning services is that they provide a choice for patients. However, it could be argued that choice could be provided within general practice and that the reason patients do not exercise a choice between GPs is because they see family planning services as providing a better service. It could therefore be argued that it would be better to improve services within general practice rather than outside it. GPs provide most of the family planning service in many areas. It is important for family planning practitioners to have a clear view of the 'public health' role they play in family planning, although, of course, training and specialist clinical expertise are some of the other important reasons for maintaining a service outside primary care.

Among the benefits to the purchaser of having an integrated purchasing plan are that it is likely to reduce the overlap of services and it is possible to request common quality standards which can be audited. It is also possible to reinforce vertical programmes by ensuring that all providers are working to a common theme.

Integrated purchasing has a number of steps (Figure 5.10). The first is to develop a strategy with providers and then to develop more detailed specifications from this strategy. This is then put out to tender. Joint work between providers and purchasers may reduce some of the problems that can be encountered during this process. Contracts may be set either directly with the main service providers or through a process of subcontracting. With subcontracting it may, for instance, be possible for a clinical directorate to purchase services which it does not supply itself from other providers, but to a specification agreed to, and audited by, the directorate.

Integrated purchasing

• Strategy
• Specification
• Tendering
• Contracts:
    Direct
    Sub-contracting

Figure 5.10

Many services within sexual health should appropriately be nurse led, both within a clinic situation and with outreach work. Specialist nurses are a key in integrating services as it is possible for them to work within and between different services. For instance, GU health advisors may well be working in family planning clinics or practice nurses may well be working both in family planning clinics or within GUM departments. This gives the potential for patients to move between services without getting 'lost' as the nurses can work on a 'named' basis caseload. For instance, if a nurse sees a patient in a family planning clinic with a vaginal discharge, she may well be able to make a direct arrangement to see her at the next convenient GUM clinic. The advantage, particularly with young people, is that the nurse is not only a friendly face but is also able to explain in some detail what investigations, examinations, etc are likely to be undertaken.

Experience with working with practice nurses shows that they may themselves refer patients from general practice to the family planning clinics within which they work, when more specialist services are needed. In addition, they may refer patients from family planning clinics back to primary care services where this is appropriate. There is great potential, even with these simple measures, to have a much more integrated service. True integration would provide a larger pool of staff able to cover the different remits of a sexual health service. Certainly it is easier to provide services, such as seven-day-a-week post-coital contraception, if there is a larger pool of people able to cover at awkward times. This may also reduce costs.

Providers have a number of choices in the way in which they can provide a more integrated service. Management structures that should be considered include bringing a variety of services together within a single clinical directorate. Where services span trusts, it may be possible for a lead clinical directorate to sub-contract for services provided by another trust. Physical structures may also encourage a more integrated approach. Accommodation is an obvious one, although some care needs to be taken in providing under a single roof services that tradition-ally have had a different image with the public. Services provided under one roof may well be appropriate in cities, but clearly, in more rural areas it is the functional integration that will be much more important than the physical integration. Ways in which integration can occur include the sharing of protocols, staff, training, quality standards and audit (Figure 5.11). Meet-ings to discuss and develop protocols and standards, etc in themselves bring together people from different disciplines to work more closely as a team.

Provider choices

- Structures
  - clinical directorate
  - accommodation
- Integration
  - shared protocols
  - shared staff
  - training
  - quality standards
  - audit

Figure 5.11

Given the pattern of need in the community and the require-ments of Government, it would appear that the time is right to develop services in a more integrated way and to begin to think of our services as sexual health services rather than as separate entities that stand alone.

References

The Health of the Nation: A Strategy for Health in England, HMSO, July, 1992.

Tackling Drugs Together: A Strategy for England 1995–1998, HMSO, May, 1995.

6 – Sexual Health Promotion in Genitourinary Medicine Clinics: Perspective of Patients

Jayshree Pillaye

Introduction

We have already heard the views of a GUM physician, a family planning doctor and a GP, and from an integrated perspective. I am going to discuss the views of a non-random sample of GUM clinic attendees who agreed to participate in a survey. This patient survey followed a quantitative study of health professionals working in GUM clinics in England. It was undertaken to identify opportunities and constraints for wider sexual health promotion in GUM clinics. The response rate to this survey was 74% (430): 76% from nurses, 73% from doctors and 71% from health advisers (Figure 6.1).

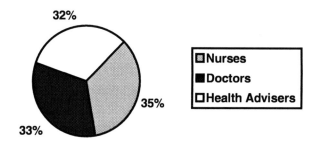

Figure 6.1   Quantity survey of health professionals

The majority (82%) responded positively when asked whether they thought that GUM clinics would be suitable for an integrated family planning and contraceptive service, whereas 25% of doctors felt that GUM clinics would be unsuitable. Some of their comments highlighted their concern for the difficulties of maintaining confidentiality, and for their limited resources:

'Poor premises and limited clinic time are the main restrictions on what health promotion can be offered in this clinic.'

There appeared to be confusion about the advantages of a separate and dedicated contraceptive service over providing an opportunistic and comprehensive service for individual patients. Some clinicians were sceptical about health promotion in a GUM clinic. They referred to the fact that funding was based upon the number of ill patients; and there was no incentive for disease prevention.

Patient Survey

This survey was undertaken to gauge patients' perception of their clinic visit, their access to information and education, and their views about a comprehensive sexual health service.

Five clinics were selected to give:

- an adequate quota of patients from the minority communities
- a varying prevalence of HIV infection and
- geographical variation

Patients were approached and asked if they would like to participate in the survey. They were given an information sheet which described the aim of the study, and were assured of confidentiality and anonymity.

A structured questionnaire was designed and patients were required to tick a Yes/No answer, with provision for comments in some questions. So as to minimise disruption to clinic routine, a single questionnaire was used for both sexes and for persons with differing sexual orientations. Piloting of the questionnaire showed that this was not problematic.

Questions covered patients' views on posters, leaflets, discussion on safer sex (including drugs and alcohol), contraception, cervical smears, perception of visit, attitude to stigma and confidentiality, and demographic data.

Results

Gender Breakdown

The total number of respondents was 511. The proportion from each clinic is shown in Figure 6.2. There were more female than male respondents.

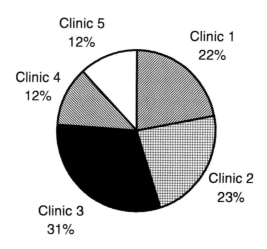

Figure 6.2   Total number of respondents

When we look at the age breakdown (Figure 6.3) it confirms both international and local findings, that most are under the age of 29. Forty one (8%) were under the age of 19. When we break these figures up further into age and gender, there are more females than males under 24 years. This pattern is similar to other studies. This is shown in Table 6.1. Black patients appeared to be over-represented and Asian groups under-represented compared to white British. Thirty four (7%) of the respondents did not answer the question on ethnicity.

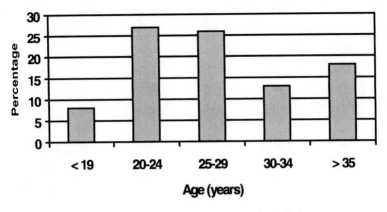

Figure 6.3   Patient survey: age breakdown

Table 6.1   Ethnicity: self-categorisation by respondents

Ethnicity	Number	Percentage
White British	308	60
White non-British	37	7
Black-Caribbean	85	17
Black-African	27	5
Indian	10	2
Pakistani	3	0.6
Bangladeshi	3	0.6
Chinese	4	0.8
Not known	34	7
Total	511	100

Posters

When asked about posters, the majority [449 (88%)] saw posters in the clinic, but many reported that the question was a prompt to look at the posters. About 1 in 5 who saw the posters said that some of the posters made them seek more information, while a small proportion [17 (3.0%)] responded that they found some of the posters upsetting.

Leaflets

Respondents were asked whether they were given any leaflets. One hundred and seventy two (34%) said they were given leaflets, with about the same proportion responding that they received some explanation about them, mainly by the doctor or nurse. Twenty-five per cent said they would have liked some written information to take away with them.

'I do suggest that there should be leaflets to read in the waiting room. It seems that only the dregs of leaflets that no one wants are left lying about.'

Homosexual men felt that the leaflets were not appropriate for them:

'I would like to know more about infections gay men can get, but all the leaflets are for heterosexual sex.'

Discussion on Safer Sex

Two hundred and sixty four (52%) responded that safer sex was discussed. Many commented that they would have liked more information.

'Not enough information, I had to ask specific questions about safer sex.'

Two hundred and eighty five (56%) reported that the use of condoms to protect against STDs and HIV was addressed. Two hundred and twenty six (44%) were offered condoms to take away, and 89 (17%) received information on how to use them, with 35 (7%) receiving information on spermicidal cream. One hundred and seventy one (34%) would have preferred more condoms, and a few commented that they would have liked more information.

'I wanted to know about condoms but they told me it was not necessary because I was getting the injection.'

Situational Factors Leading to Unsafe Sex

The respondents were asked about situational factors that may lead to unsafe sex. Ninety four (18%) reported that drugs as a factor leading to unsafe sex was discussed, while 64 (13%) said that alcohol was discussed. Sixty five (13%) were advised about Hepatitis B vaccine.

Contraception

Respondents were asked whether contraception was discussed with them. One hundred and seventy seven (38%) of all respondents reported that contraception was discussed; 67% of these were female. Two hundred and nineteen (50% – two thirds females) stated that discussion of contraception would be relevant for them at a GUM clinic. Two hundred and thirty seven (62%) would find it more convenient to get this advice at a GUM clinic; 60% of them were women.

Two hundred and seven (41%) said they would go to their GP for follow-up contraception; 147 (29%) said they would go to the family planning clinic for follow up, and the same proportion were unsure where they would go for follow-up advice for contraception.

One hundred and eleven (22%) said they would be embarrassed to tell their GP that they attended the GUM clinic, and 76 (15%) said they would be embarrassed to tell their FP clinic.

Prophylaxis

The question regarding prevention of unintended pregnancies (Figure 6.4) showed that about 79 (22%) would use condoms alone and 96 (26%) the pill alone, 128 (35%) condoms and the pill, 23 (6%) condom and spermicide, and 28 (11%) other methods.

When asked how they would avoid both STDs and pregnancies, 178 (49%) responded that they would use the condom and the pill, 127 (35%) would use condoms alone, 33 (9%) condoms and spermicide, and 20 (6%) other methods. Four (1%) reported that they would use the pill alone (Figure 6.4).

Some felt that the questions on contraception and prophylaxis were irrelevant for them because they were either sterilised or had an IUD inserted, or were receiving Depo-Provera injections.

Emergency Contraception

One hundred and fifty seven (47%) of women knew about emergency contraception, but only 43 (13%) of men responded that they did not know about it. One hundred and four (41%) were aware they could obtain it from their GP, 72 (28%) from the FP clinic and only 29 (11%) from GUM clinics.

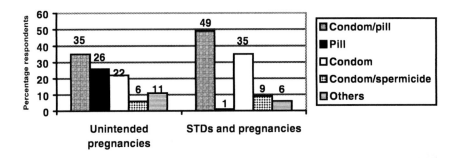

Figure 6.4   Results of the question on the prevention of unintended pregnancy and STD

Cervical Smears

Two hundred and five (74%) women reported that cervical smears were discussed with them, and 14 (5%) women reported that they have never had a smear. Just under half of the women [130 (49%)] would have liked more information about cervical neoplasia.

Some of the comments confirmed poor knowledge about cervical screening.

> *'What can be found out with a smear? Example – AIDS. Or do you have to have an additional test?'*

Fifty seven per cent had their smears at the GP, 14% at the GUM clinic and 7% at the FP clinic; 20% had had a smear at more than one of these clinics, and only 2% at the gynaecology or antenatal clinic (Figure 6.5).

When asked where they would like to have their smears taken, 42% preferred to have it taken at the GUM clinic, 39% at their GP, 12% at the FP clinic and 7% did not mind having it taken at any of these clinics (Figure 6.5).

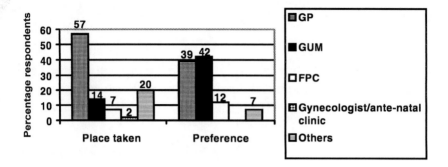

Figure 6.5

General Comments

Three hundred and ninety five (77%) found the information and discussion at the clinic useful, with 264 (52%) reporting that some of the information was new and 70% reporting that the information made things clearer. Many, however, also commented that they wanted more information.

> *'Herpes, cervical cancer, tests. I did not know anything about tests or why they were taken, they just took them.'*

Safer Sex

Two hundred and fifty eight (51%) reported that they would use a condom every time, and 338 (66%) would use a condom with new partners. Three hundred and one (59%) said they would avoid sex if they did not have condoms.

HIV Infection

Two hundred (47%) said no one discussed HIV infection with them. Ninety four (22%) reported that HIV was discussed by the doctor, 14% by the health adviser, and 8% by the nurse, and 9% reported that a combination of those three professionals discussed it with them. Twenty (4%) said they were offended by staff talking about HIV to them, and 88% that they would be comfortable talking about HIV and AIDS with clinic staff.

For a few, HIV and AIDS appeared to instil a great anxiety.

'AIDS and HIV just freaks me out.'

'One big fear – I would rather not know. I will not have a test.'

Perception of Visit

Three hundred and ninety two (77%) said they were comfortable with the receptionist, nurse, doctor and health adviser; and four hundred and thirty five (85%) reported that they believed these professionals were comfortable with them. However, a high proportion [256 (50%)] recorded that they did not see a health adviser.

Many more commented that they wanted to know what would happen to them when they attended a GUM clinic, and wanted to know why they had to see so many people. Many were also unhappy that they spent so long at the clinic even when they had made appointments.

Stigma

Patients were given a series of statements and they were required to state how strongly they agreed or disagreed with each.

One hundred and thirty five (28%) strongly disagreed, and 29 (6%) strongly agreed that the GUM clinic should inform their GP about this visit.

One hundred and twenty three (27%) strongly disagreed, and 18 (4%) strongly agreed that the GUM clinic should inform the FP clinic about this visit. Two hundred and forty two (50%) strongly agreed that people should not feel ashamed to attend a GUM clinic, and 6 (1%) strongly disagreed and 261 (54%) strongly agreed that they should get all their sexual health promotion, tests and treatment at the GUM clinic. No one strongly disagreed.

'People should not feel ashamed, but they do. The general image to most people is a place where people come to get rid of the clap. Can anything be done to improve this?'

Seventy two (15%) strongly agreed, and 60 (13%) strongly disagreed that the name *GUM clinic* should be changed to *Sexual Health Clinic*; 137 (29%) were uncertain – 110 (23%) agreed and

20% disagreed. Many added comments that the name was irrelevant.

> '*It makes no odds what it is called, it's the social inhibition that's the problem.*'

Discussion

This and other surveys confirm that more young people, especially young women, were attending GUM clinics, and that pregnancy and STDs were a major concern. The needs of women who were at risk of pregnancy and STDs are often the same.

This patient survey showed that many patients did not receive leaflets, information on contraception and information on HIV infection. Many women commented that they wanted more information on cervical cancer and colposcopy. Some of the reasons that patients may not have received counselling and patient education include:

- many of these patients did not see a health adviser, although it was presumed that they had
- patients who came for specific treatments (warts, colposcopy) bypassed the 'routine' procedures
- health professionals did not think it was necessary, or felt uncomfortable
- lack of time by clinic staff and patients

Some patients remarked that they were not asked about their partner's sexual lifestyle. Other patients remarked that on previous occasions they did not return for results and treatment because of the long waiting time on their first visit. Patient compliance appears to be affected by accessibility and convenience of clinic waiting and opening times.

All the clinics visited had supplies of oral contraception and provided an emergency contraceptive service. Yet only 11% of the patients surveyed knew they could obtain postcoital contraception from their GUM clinic. Just less than half the patients surveyed were offered condoms, and about 45% would have preferred more condoms. A few health professionals remarked that they did not hand out condoms because patients were advised to refrain from sexual intercourse until their treatment was complete.

There appears to be some reluctance on the part of health professionals to advocate dual protection for STDs and pregnancy (condom + pill = 'double Dutch'). However, patients in this sample were already taking this on board. Thirty five per cent said they would use the condom and pill to prevent pregnancy, and 49% that they would use both methods to protect against both STDs and pregnancy. It therefore appears a method acceptable to people at risk of STDs and unplanned pregnancy, and should be encouraged.

Men who identified themselves as gay felt they were receiving inadequate information on safer sex and wanted more discussion and information. Some described clinic leaflets as 'heterosexist'. They themselves admitted to no unease in attending a GUM clinic, but a few felt that some doctors were not so comfortable with them.

Clinic attenders identifying themselves as being from the minority ethnic population appear to be over-represented in this sample. However, the clinics were selected to give an adequate quota from the minority population. There is considerable variation within minority ethnic communities. Black-Caribbeans and Africans appear to be over-represented, while south Asians and Chinese are under-represented. Further monitoring and surveillance is needed to collaborate these findings, and to ascertain reasons for this. Black-Caribbean and African communities may be attending GUM clinics in preference to accessing other services (GP, FP clinics). Anecdotal reports support the findings that Asians are not accessing GUM services. There is a need for further information and education about STDs targeted to these communities, and for services to be made culturally appropriate and sensitive.

Summary and Conclusion

GUM clinics have an important public health role of prevention and education. Other studies have shown that there is some difficulty in deciding on the 'trade off' between the treatment of individuals and the public health role of prevention and education. There appeared to be no systematic way of providing information on primary prevention for the individual clinic attendee, or for their sexual partners.

Many patients did not know what to expect on their first visit, and could not distinguish between the health professionals working in a GUM clinic. They wanted more information about who they were going to see, the reasons for tests being done, and how long they were likely to spend at the clinic.

The patients interviewed wished to receive sexual health promotion at their GUM clinic visit. However, there still appeared to be some stigma attached to attending a GUM clinic, and clinic attenders did not wish others, including their GP, to know about their visit. But, although acknowledging the stigma, they did not feel it should be a barrier to wider sexual health promotion once they actually attend the clinic.

Combining STD prevention and treatment, prevention of unintended pregnancies and promoting sexual health makes medical, social and economic sense.

7 – Risk Taking and Safer Sex: Are They Irreconcilable?

Helen Ward

Introduction

A friend of mine is part of a consortium at work where they buy 10 National Lottery tickets each week. One week she missed the draw on television, and didn't know whether she had won. On hearing that that the jackpot of around £10 000 000 was likely to be shared by several people, she said, 'it would be just my luck to win this week when the jackpot is small'. This may seem a long way from sexual health, but I have introduced the example of Gill's gambling as a reminder of some broader attitudes to risk and risk taking. Millions of people buy their £1 lottery tickets each week and are almost certain to lose the money; it is a very 'risky' activity. But the millions of people continue to place their bets. They do it because taking this risk produces the possibility, albeit about 13 000 000:1 against, of making a large gain. What Gill expressed was first that she thought, incorrectly, that if she won this week she would have less chance of winning the following week, and second, that she wanted the gain to be considerable, not just the odd £10 000. She wanted the risk she took to be worth it. In this paper I look briefly at different concepts of risk, provide examples of how risk is discussed in the sex industry, and then show how a broader understanding of risk may help to focus health promotion on particular individuals and groups. I am assuming a shared objective of promoting safer sex through risk reduction rather than promoting the avoidance of sex *per se*. The main message is that shifting sexual behaviour in ways that may reduce adverse health outcomes cannot simply be achieved through the giving of information about risks. Indeed, posed in a generally negative way, information on safer sex is likely to convey an anti-sex message which will not be accepted by many who could benefit, including younger people and those whose behaviour is already condemned by much of society, for example, people with multiple sexual partners, prostitutes, and gay men.

Concepts of Risk

Medical

In the health field we tend to equate risk with danger and adverse events; indeed that is how risk is generally understood. For epidemiologists risk has a very precise meaning:

> '... the probability that an event will occur, e.g. that an individual will become ill or die within a stated period of time or age.'

(Last[1])

The event of interest is almost always disease or death, and risk therefore has wholly negative connotations. The objective of epidemiological research is generally to identify factors that are associated with increased risk in the hope that we can then eliminate those that are susceptible to intervention, and thus reduce the burden of disease and death. But many such risks are the result of individual or social action: climbing a mountain, building a factory to process chemicals, designing low-cost housing, taking drugs such as alcohol or tobacco, having sex. People do not set out to break their legs when they visit the ski slopes, but it is more likely to happen there than if they stayed at home. Skiing therefore increases the risk of a broken limb, just as smoking increases the risk of lung cancer. In neither case is the disease the objective of the action. The health risks associated with some of these activities are generally unwanted by-products. For these reasons, knowledge of health risks is not enough on its own to alter most actions and behaviours.

In 1983 John Ashton[2], a leading public health physician, wrote:

'As a species we are risk taking animals, but we resent risks being imposed upon us by others. We like to feel in control, and most people are much more worried by flying than by driving their own car or riding a bicycle – even though car drivers are six times, and cyclists 60 times, more likely to be killed than passengers on a scheduled airline.'

Gambling

The medical understanding of risk, largely negative, is not the only one. In the seventeenth century the concept of risk was first associated with gambling: a specialised mathematical analysis of chance was developed[3]. Risk then meant the probability of an event occurring, combined with the magnitude of the losses or gains that would occur. The negative outcome was only one part of the risk calculation – risk was more of a cost–benefit analysis.

Since the seventeenth century the analysis of probabilities has become the basis of scientific knowledge, transforming the nature of evidence, of knowledge, of authority and of logic. Any process or activity has its probabilities of success or failure. The calculation of risk is deeply entrenched in science and manufacturing, and as a theoretical basis for decision making. Clearly, the probability theory has provided a modern way of thinking.

Risk analysis in general can be thought to encompass not only danger, but also potential gain. In some spheres risk is not seen in the negative way familiar to us. Nick Leeson is believed to have lost Barings Bank over £750 000 000 through his dabblings on the futures market. He did it through taking risks, but, presumably, his aim was not to lose any money, but rather to make money through taking risks. If things had gone better for him he would have been a modern capitalist hero. Indeed risk taking is a fundamental part of entrepreneurial capitalism; waged workers are paid for their labour power for a specific period of time; the entrepreneurs receive higher incomes, justified on the basis of their greater risk, a threat realised when they occasionally go spectacularly bankrupt.

Sin and Taboo

Mary Douglas[3] has written extensively on risk. She compares the role of the modern concept of risk to that of concepts of sin and taboo in more religious societies. While risk is scientific and thereby 'neutral', it can be used to arrive at an apparent consensus view of acceptable actions. Those who do not follow these norms then place themselves, and others, 'at risk'.

This may help to explain the debate that emerged in the 1980s over the use of the term 'risk group' in relation to HIV and AIDS. The definition of gay men, injecting drug users or people from sub-Saharan Africa as risk groups for HIV/AIDS was broadly rejected first by rights activists and then by health workers, as it was felt to generalise, and add to, existing stigma. The term came from epidemiological studies which group people according to various characteristics to look at associations and thereby generate hypotheses about the aetiology and natural history of disease. Classical methods for investigation of any disease start with defining who is affected by person, time and place – who got it, when and where. This is then extended to groups; men, for example, are at greater risk of cardiovascular disease than women. They could be called a 'high risk group'. Not all men get cardio-vascular disease, and further investigation may narrow down who, within that broad group, is at risk – those who smoke, who have hypertension, or who are overweight, for example. As more is understood about the pathogenesis and epidemiology of diseases we can be more and more specific about categorising people's risks of disease as groups or as individuals. Until greater precision in prediction is achieved, the need to group people to indicate relative risks of disease will remain.

The underlying objection to the term 'high risk group' for AIDS was that it was applied to already stigmatised and oppressed groups (gay men, drug injectors, prostitutes, migrants, poor people) and there was fear that it would intensify the oppression. However, by avoiding the identification of increased risk of disease with pre-existing oppression and stigma, this may have led to a denial, or concealment, of the role that the oppression itself had in creating that increased risk. More recently, there have been calls for a 're-gaying' of AIDS, a recognition that in the UK and similar countries, gay men are worst hit, and their needs as a group and as individuals are not being met.

> *'The danger of contagion was employed to justify the new social policies of sixteenth century municipalities ... the isolation procedures taken against the plague would not have been so savage if the poor had not presented a conscious target which was subject to attack for other reasons. It is significant that plague regulations were most clearly and strictly formulated when the socially discriminatory disease became conspicuous.'*
>
> (Slack[4])

Fear of danger, as in response to a new epidemic, tends to strengthen the lines of division in a community. Rejecting the term 'risk group' was an attempt to prevent the new plague of AIDS being used to intensify existing oppression. The result is to focus more on the individual – the term 'high risk behaviour group' was suggested – with the consequent danger of apportionment of blame to these individuals, itself with the consequent denial of rights or access to support. This twentieth century individualism leads to the neglect of the role of social relations in explaining health risks. The increased risk of HIV in gay men in general can be explained by the social position of gay men as much as by their individual 'high risk behaviours'; similarly the higher mortality of the unemployed can be explained by poverty as much as by the fact that they have poorer diet or smoke too much.

Recognition of the existence of groups who are at increased risk as a result of their role in society has the advantage of suggesting the potential for organising a collective resistance to the threat (of disease and stigma).

The fact that there was a pre-existing visible gay community has done much to assist the fight against AIDS. Other groups that are less visible and more atomised – drug users, migrants – have more difficulty.

An individualist culture finds ways of making its disadvantaged members disappear from sight. Cultural analysis is a countervailing vision which warns what categories in each kind of culture are most likely to be at risk, who will be sinned against and who will be counted as the sinner exposing the others to risk. It is true, as Charles Rosenburg says, that:

'Cultural values and social location have always provided the materials for self-serving constructions of epidemiological risk. The poor, the alien, the sinner have all served as convenient objects for such stigmatising speculations.'

(Douglas[3])

Concepts of Risk – Prostitutes and their Sexual Partners

Risk is therefore understood differently according to your perspective – some see it as a way of analysing distribution of disease and its determinants, some as a way of making decisions about action, others as a way of apportioning blame.

In work that we have carried out at St Mary's Hospital over the past nine years with female sex workers and their sexual partners, risk has not surprisingly been a recurring theme. Risk was central to the agenda of researchers and health care workers – measuring risk and known risk factors for HIV and STD, finding ways to help reduce that risk, and so on. Since 1986 I have carried out clinical and epidemiological research in this field alongside Sophie Day, an anthropologist. During the research we talked to men and women about their understanding of risk, their own risks and their strategies for dealing with this. There was no need to ask specific questions on risk in interviews with prostitutes. Records of discussions in the clinic, and transcripts of more- and less-structured interviews, reveal that risk was a constant theme.

Prostitutes

Women we talked to between 1986 and 1988 were very fearful of AIDS, raising questions about the degree of risk from their work in general and risks from particular forms of contact (oral sex, kissing, masturbation, water sports, sex during menstruation, etc). Women talked explicitly about the risks and about their attempts to minimise them. Condom use for vaginal sex with clients increased dramatically in these years[5]). Prostitutes had used condoms for commercial sex in the past, but this became far more consistent. Condoms had to be used not only for vaginal intercourse but also for oral sex and even for masturbation. Anal sex was less and less commonly reported. Fewer clients were exempted from these general rules – in the past, regulars and other 'good' clients would be allowed unprotected sex by some women. This became rare by the late 1980s.

Other risk-reduction measures were introduced or made more systematic. One woman reported that clients were also more concerned about safety:

> *'The clients are really concerned now ... they inspect the beds and the bathroom, insist on clean towels after every client, inspect the lavatory. It's strange, they never used to be so conscientious. Most of them are married, a lot of them are scared to have sex – one geezer came last week said he didn't want to have sex, he wouldn't mind trying domination but he was frightened of that too. In the end he said "I think its better if I go back to my own missus and have sex with her, or at least try sex with her", so he went away again, I can't blame him.... A lot of them check me out, saying do I do oral, do I do anal, do I use contraceptives, have I been with anyone else, and then they say they'll offer me money and I say no, no, no and then in the end they say they were just checking me out.'*

Many women reported using more than one condom, using spermicidal pessaries, creams, foams and sponges. Women obtained special douches from abroad 'to prevent infections' – these were from France and Germany, and one woman got them specially from Brazil. Oral sex, with or without condoms, was followed by mouthwashing – this was never information we explicitly sought, but a number of women reported using Listerine and other substances as mouthwashes, Dettol in the bath, vinegar in the vagina, chlorhexidine for hand washing, surgical gloves – some women sounded as if they followed better infection control procedures than we have in hospitals!

For these women, risk reduction makes sense. This is work, and risk of disease is an occupational hazard. Decisions about risk taking are based on a more or less explicit balancing of possible outcomes – gains and losses.

Looked at from this perspective, risk fits in well with the business ethic of the prostitutes we talked to. Business is done on the basis of a system of costs and benefits: risks are a hazard, profit is the motive. Considering the exchanges in this way, it is not surprising that prostitutes as entrepreneurs are, in general, very good consumers of health promotion messages. In business you maximise gain and minimise costs, and these are explicitly addressed in the negotiation. Sexual services are costed, safety insisted upon and terms agreed.

The importance of looking at risk behaviour in context is shown by the contrast in prostitutes' private sexual relations[6,7]. Condoms are rarely used for non-commercial sex, even where the partner is known to be 'risky', i.e. a previous source of an STD, or someone with many other partners. This distinction between commercial and non-commercial sex and associated risks is now well established[8]. But it serves to reinforce the point that the same women who are meticulous at reducing their risk in one setting, who are highly knowledgeable and have access to all the necessary resources, will take great risks in another setting.

Prostitutes argue that condoms and other forms of risk reduction cannot be introduced into their private sexual lives as this would signify 'business' to them. Unfortunately as business goes out of the window, so does safety for many women. This creates a problem for risk reduction strategies for prostitutes: the more risk reduction messages are associated with good business practice, the more difficult it is to introduce them into a relationship based on intimacy and passion.

Clients of Prostitutes

When the first government advertisements on AIDS went out in 1987, prostitutes reported a major impact on clients. Clients were worried and more open to discussing risks of infection and to accepting the need to use condoms. This is not universal of course, but serves to show that clients are also concerned. We carried out interviews with approximately a hundred clients of female prostitutes in 1990–91[9]. They were indeed concerned about risks of HIV and other STDs, but tended to talk about it in a different way. They were concerned about catching an infection that they might pass on to another partner. A number of men reported that they no longer went to prostitutes because of fear of AIDS. AIDS is seen as a much greater problem that other STDs.

> *'Comparing the risk of STD to AIDS is like comparing the risk of coal to that of nuclear power stations.'*

> *'I don't worry about STDs from casual partners ... there is a risk but it isn't a great risk like driving on the M1.'*

Interestingly, some clients also said they had offered women more for sex without a condom to 'test them out' (as reported by the prostitute quoted above), and if they agreed, deciding that the woman was not safe. Many said they avoided prostitutes who they thought may be at increased risk:

> *'I would never go to one on drugs ... I can tell by their eyes and their mannerisms.'*

> *'I avoid ones that don't look particularly well, such as people using drugs, pale complexion, shallow eyes. I'd avoid drug users because of fear of AIDS, I don't want to infect others or myself.'*

One man reported avoiding situations where he might go to a prostitute when he was not in full possession of his faculties, as

> *'I might take risks with my own health; I'd also avoid environments like dirty flat or stairwell.'*

These men can be seen to have similar concerns as the prostitutes, and take steps to reduce risk. However, they do not have identical interests in the situation, as they are not involved in a purely commercial transaction. When they talked about why they went to prostitutes, various motivations were expressed. Of importance to our work are comments such as these:

> *'the seedy nature, its more exciting'*

> *'its a thrill ... dangerous but not lethal'*

> *'looking for risks'*

> *'its exciting to pay for sex'*

These comments show that, for some clients at least, the risk involved in going to a prostitute is part of the enjoyment. Most people will remember when a senior member of the justice system, at the time Director of Public Prosecutions, was arrested for kerb crawling in King's Cross. We can't be sure, but there must have been a large element of playing with risk in his actions. Whatever psychological, social or political interpretations can be put on that particular case, the general issue of a positive image of risk taking has to be addressed in developing sexual health programmes.

Several clients volunteered the opinion that there should be some regulation:

> *'There should be screening for STDs and AIDS; it would be better if it was legalised, with women available who were clean.'*

> *'There should be medical services like there are in Las Vegas where prostitutes have regular check ups once a month.'*

> *'Its better in Holland where they're cleaner, more regulated, ... no fear, no shame or risk.'*

That suggests that some men would prefer the state to provide them with a 'clean' supply of prostitutes, and then they can enjoy the thrill of being wicked, i.e. the risk of being frowned upon, without taking the risk of getting a serious infection.

One man had been able to link the two apparently counterposed approaches to risk – appealing to the concern for risk reduction through condom use, and also appealing to the clients' desire to take a risk by having sex with a prostitute:

> *'There's something addictive about using condoms with prostitutes. Or maybe its because of the association of condoms and prostitutes – a bit like the difference between sex with your wife and sex with a prostitute. They can be associated with the naughty side and be quite exciting, even if sensation is reduced and you can't linger.'*

If only we could convince all clients, and others who enjoy taking risks, to identify condoms with being naughty!

Approaches to Modifying Risk

This brief presentation of results highlights a central issue: people do not have a static concept of risk which is applicable to all contexts.

Understanding possible risks and ways of reducing them informs decision making, but many other factors affect those decisions. From the perspective of planning health services and particularly health promotion activities, these insights may be useful in tailoring messages. The government has set targets that focus on young people. Unfortunately for us, as Widdus *et al.*[10] point out:

> *'Adolescents seems to have a sense of personal invulnerability and immortality, and a propensity for risk seeking and risk taking.'*

We need to recognise that decisions about sexual activity are not taken simply on the basis of rational cost–benefit assessments, least of all by those who are young and inexperienced.

We have basic responsibilities to ensure that people are educated about the possibilities of infection and pregnancy, and in how these risks can be minimised. We can provide condoms and contraception, and training in negotiating safer sex. But if our messages to young people are to be successful we have to think about how they approach risk and the way they think about sex. Unfortunately, sex is frequently seen as something that young people are not supposed to do, that it is naughty and rebellious to do it. Most young people have to be inventive in finding places and times to have sex, and it is shrouded in secrecy and deceit. These are not the most favourable conditions in which to promote rational decision making about safer sex.

It has been suggested that we should focus not on high risk groups or even behaviours, but on high risk situations for preventing AIDS transmission[11]. This includes situations such as large scale migration and urbanisation, and war. But this can equally apply to less dramatic situations, including where alcohol or other drugs are used, where opportunities for casual sex are greater (such as holidays, business travel, conferences).

Rose[12] wrote that:

> *'People are generally motivated only by the prospect of a benefit which is visible, early, and likely.'*

Young people in particular may be less likely to be motivated by fears of something that might happen in 10 to 15 years time than what their peers will think tomorrow. This provides openings for risk reduction which concentrate on social groups and situations rather than individuals. I fear that all too often health promotion is seen as yet another set of worthy adults trying to constrain the behaviour of youth. If that is the case with sexual health then we may have as little success as we seem to be having in relation to young women and smoking. Innovative methods are being developed using peer group education, positive images of sex for young people, and generally promoting choice to have better sex rather than appearing to be passion-killers.

References

1. Last, J. M. (1988). *A Dictionary of Epidemiology*. OUP, New York, 2nd edn.
2. Ashton, J. R. (1983). Risk Assessment. *BMJ*, **286**, 1843.
3. Douglas, M. (1990). Risk as a forensic resource. *Daedalus*, **119**(4), 1–16.
4. Slack, P. (1988). *Responses to Plague*. Quoted in Douglas (1990), *ibid.*
5. Day, S. and Ward, H. (1990). The Praed Street Project: a cohort of prostitute women in London. In *AIDS, Drugs and Prostitution*. (Ed. Plant, M.), Routledge, London.
6. Day, S., Ward, H. and Harris, J. R. W. (1988). Prostitute women and public health. *BMJ*, **297**, 1585.
7. Ward, H., Day, S., Mezzone, J., Dunlop, L., Donegan, C., Farrar, S., Whitaker, L., Harris, J. R. W. and Miller, D. L. (1993). Prostitution and risk of HIV: female prostitutes in London. *BMJ*, **307**, 356–358.
8. Mak, R. (Ed.) (1996). *European Project for AIDS Prevention in Prostitution*, Academic Press.
9. Day, S., Ward, H. and Perrotta, L. (1993). Prostitution and risk of HIV: male partners of female prostitutes. *BMJ*, **307**, 359–361.
10. Widdus, R., Meheus, A. and Short, R. (1990). The management of risk in sexually transmitted diseases. *Daedalus*, **119**, 177–191.
11. Zwi, A. B. and Cabral, A. J. R. (1991). Identifying 'high risk situations' for preventing AIDS. *BMJ*, **303**, 1527–1529.
12. Rose, G. (1992). *The Strategy of Preventive Medicine*, OUP, Oxford.

Section 2

Reports from the Workgroups

8 – Workgroup 1: Components for Future Purchasing

Purchasing Priorities, Resource Allocation and Contracting

Sarah Randall

Group Facilitator: *Peter Bellamy*

Group Rapporteur: *Sarah Randall*

The remit for this group was to discuss the components for future purchasing and included purchasing priorities, resource allocation and contracting for the provision of services regarding all aspects of sexual health.

The group had a wide ranging discussion on aspects of good practice in relation to sexual and reproductive health in its widest concept and made four recommendations.

Recommendations

1. *To protect and strengthen the public health by maintaining provision of free sexual health services (STD + contraception + health promotion) to which people can refer themselves, and which are appropriate and responsive to local needs.*

This recommendation ensures that there is a safety net and an element of choice for those people who do not, for whatever reason, want to attend primary health care services, i.e. their general practitioner or practice nurse. It also ensures that there is provision for those individuals who are not registered with a general practitioner and will include various 'at risk' groups, for example, the homeless, travellers and some immigrants.

The self-referral element was deemed to be important as it allows people to access the service without first having to obtain a letter of referral, and they can attend where and when it is convenient to them. They do not necessarily have to attend a clinic near to where they live.

Contact tracing is an important part of GUM services and helps to ensure that untreated and asymptomatic STDs are treated and managed appropriately.

Improving and providing easy access were felt to be important in reducing unplanned pregnancies.

To achieve this recommendation, it was agreed that purchasers should provide the following:

- STD care and control
- Prevention of unplanned pregnancies
- Sexual health promotion
- HIV prevention and care

2. Development of specialist sexual health services by the convergence of family planning and genitourinary medicine services

This would ensure that people using services have access to an appropriate range of care at one time, in response to expressed wishes. It could reduce unnecessary multiple attendances and conserve resources. It may also help clients to overcome their reluctance to attend some GUM services which they may still associate with the 'VD' or 'clap' clinic.

Obviously arrangements for convergence would vary depending on local situations.

The current structure of services often results in unmet needs for contraceptive care in GUM and unmet STD needs in FP clinics. In particular it was felt that access to emergency contraception could be widened by GUM also offering this service.

3. Purchasers should consider ways in which primary care interfaces and receives support from these specialist services.

It was appreciated that primary health care providers need access to advice and referral to secondary specialist services. There may be shared guidelines and audit across the interface and the specialist services may be able to provide training for primary health care staff to improve the quality of their services.

4. It is not anticipated that these recommendations will need extra resources.

The group reckoned that by working together, GUM and FP services could offer a total package greater than the sum of each individual service. However, practically, it was recognised that the outcome would vary considerably between districts dependent on current service provision and strategic plans that were already being implemented by health authorities and trusts. It was felt that total GP fundholding and other aspects of commissioning services could affect provision of care, but the group felt they were not in a position to discuss this aspect further.

In conclusion, the group wished the outcomes of the conference, and especially the consensus statement, to be widely distributed.

9 – Collaboration Between Genitourinary Medicine and Family Planning

A. B. Alawattegama and Helen Massil

Group Facilitators: *Jennifer Wordsworth and Penny Chandiok*

Group Rapporteurs: *Anura Alawattegama and Helen Massil*

Introduction

The specialties of GUM and FP are concerned with promoting sexual health and well-being by encouraging positive aspects of sexual health through good personal and sexual relationships, and by reducing the negative or adverse outcomes of sexual activity, such as unwanted pregnancies and the acquisition of sexually transmitted diseases (STDs) including human immunodeficiency virus (HIV). For these reasons HIV/AIDS, STDs and sexual health (including family planning and contraception) were identified, along with drug misuse, as 'key areas' in *The Health of the Nation*[1]. Although the emphasis of GUM and FP services may be somewhat different, the sexual behaviour of women attending either service appears to be the same[2].

Of the three major agencies within the NHS providing specific sexual health services, GUM and FP specialties have in common open access, self-referral and are free of charge. However, traditionally the specialities have developed independently, each speciality focusing on and emphasising different elements of sexual health without considering the impact of one on the other[3,4].

Women with sexual health problems are most likely to present to FP or GUM clinics. However, those attending FP services mainly request contraception, but overtly or covertly have concerns regarding STDs, while those attending GUM services require contraception, although their primary concern may be to exclude an STD. These women have male partners who rarely attend FP services and may attend a GUM clinic.

Family planning focuses on prevention of pregnancies, and GUM focuses on treatment and prevention of genital infection with some overlap occurring, depending on available expertise and facilities. This fragmented approach to health care may result in incomplete or inappropriate provision for the sexual health needs of the individual attending any one of the specialities.

Working Together

The advantages of integrated health care under one roof have been elaborated[5,6]. However, in developing such an approach, consideration should be given to the local needs, available expertise and differing career structures and training. Such services should be innovative to local needs and provider designed, and led through a forum consisting of providers from which an agreed leadership will develop an appropriately integrated sexual health service. Involvement of purchasers at an early stage may not be appropriate, or indeed may be detrimental to the development of an integrated sexual health strategy if the providers do not have an agreed approach.

Another model is to set up a working group to establish contact between both specialities, with the opportunity to bring in other interested agencies such as general practice and public health representatives.

Collaboration between GUM and FP services should be the minimum aim, while some services will choose to be fully integrated. To develop such a strategy, providers of GUM and FP services should be aware of each other's services, their own limitations and have mutual respect for each other's expertise. Additionally, since improving and promoting sexual health involve other agencies and organisations, such as Brook, British Pregnancy Advisory Service (BPAS) and Pregnancy Advisory Service (PAS), with differing but complementary roles, it may be appropriate to include these agencies in developing sexual health strategies appropriate to the community. Such a participative strategy will increase collaboration between the different agencies by overcoming barriers, creating synergy and common ownership, and avoiding un- necessary duplication, and will enhance education of purchasers of health care to protect and develop sexual health services appropriate to local needs.

Appropriate Referral Between Services

Appropriate referral between services should be facilitated by identi- fying within each locality or community the main access points for contraceptive, STD and sexual health advice and ensuring that these are linked to the source of expertise. The services should be avail- able to all who are considering sexual activity and those who are sexually active, but should also target people at greatest risk or with special needs. Thus the range of choices and the routes of access should be made clear to each provider and service user. Adequate information on clinic times, contact telephone numbers, com- munication lines and a list of expertise should also be available to each provider. It is desirable that both GUM and FP are aware of, and advertise, each other's services widely.

In providing advice, risk assessment is essential, as the most effective contraceptive method preventing transmission of STDs may be the least effective in providing contraception, and, conversely, the most effective contraceptive methods may be the least effective for preventing transmission of STDs. Indeed, some methods of contraception may increase the risk of acquisition or complications of STDs. Therefore both services need to be able to undertake risk assessments by means of sexual and contraceptive histories, to enable appropriate referral or consultation between services. Where staff lack such skills, joint service training should be undertaken. In developing such referral systems, arrangements need to be made to ensure that patients are not lost 'in transit' and that adequate contact tracing takes place. An interface audit, undertaken in south-east London, between a family planning service (FPS) and five local GUM services, demonstrated that only 52.7% of women referred with a positive or equivocal *Chlamydia* result actually attended a GUM clinic. The average time from test to referral was 15.8 days (5–111), while average time from referral to attendance at a GUM clinic was 12 days (1–86)[7]. This audit was undertaken in a deprived inner city area, with high rates of sexually transmitted diseases and a very mobile population. In contrast, a similar audit was conducted in south Manchester between one family planning and one genitourinary medicine service. The audit found that 86% of referred women from the family planning service attended the local GUM clinic and attendance rose to 96% after careful follow up[8]. This audit was undertaken in a relatively affluent, stable population (compared to that in south-east London) and was simplified by the involvement of one FPS and a single GUM service. The results from both these audits demonstrate the importance of establishing the needs of the local population and undertaking appropriate management. Additionally, communication between the two specialities should be improved to inform each other of the outcome of referrals. The use of health advisors as a source of link between the specialities will enable the setting up of 'fail safe' systems.

Joint Protocols

Certain groups of clients have been demonstrated to be at higher risk of STDs[9]. Such groups include clients under 25 years of age and women requesting a termination of pregnancy. Services could work on joint protocols to reduce the risk of pelvic inflammatory disease (PID) associated with such groups of women, possibly in association with the local health authority. The RCOG recently published recommendations for antibiotic prophylaxis and/or screening for sexually transmitted infections prior to termination of pregnancy[10]. Joint protocols will also facilitate appropriate referral.

Interface Audits

Interface audits provide valuable information on how well services are performing and identify areas for improvement. However, interface audits will not be successful unless all services are actively involved and prepared to make appropriate changes when identified. Some examples of interface audits include:

- Clients referred from FP services to GUM services with a positive *Chlamydia* result.
- Clients referred from GUM services to FP services for on-going contraception provision.
- Clients requesting a termination of pregnancy, identified to have a sexually transmitted disease.

Conclusion

Collaboration between family planning and genitourinary medicine services can range from formal discussions to ensure more appropriate referral and working practices, to full integration. The decision will depend on local population needs. However, there is a wealth of opportunities to ensure that working practices are improved and that both specialities provide efficient and effective services for clients.

References

1. Department of Health (1992). *The Health of the Nation: A strategy for Health in England*, Cm 1986, HMSO, London (ISBN 0101198620).
2. Radcliffe, K. W., Tasker, T., Evans, B. A., Bispham, A. and Snelling, M. (1993). A comparison of sexual behaviour and risk behaviour between women in three clinical settings. *Genitourin. Med.*, **69**, 441–445.
3. Cates, W. Jr and Stone, C. (1992). Family planning – sexually transmitted diseases and contraceptive choice: a literature update. Part 1. *Fam. Plan. Perspect.*, **24**(2), 75–84.
4. Cates, W. Jr and Stone, C. (1992). Family planning – sexually transmitted diseases and contraceptive choice: a literature update. Part 2. *Fam. Plan. Perspect.*, **24**(3), 122–8.

5. Greenhouse, P. (1994). A sexual health service under one roof: setting up sexual health services for women. *J. Mat. Child Health*, **19**, 228–233.

6. Stedman, Y and Elstein, M. (1995). Rethinking sexual health clinics. *Br. Med. J.*, **310**, 342–343.

7. Wilkinson, C. and Massil, H. (1996). Interface audit of *Chlamydia* screening in community family planning clinics and referral to genito-urinary clinics. Fourth Congress of the European Society of Contraception, Barcelona.

8. Sin, J., Gbolade, B. A., Russell, A., Chandiok, P. and Kirkman, R. E. (1996). Referral compliance of *Chlamydia* positive patients from a family planning clinic. *Br. J. Family Planning*, **22**, 155–156.

9. Fish, A. N., Fairweather, D. V., Oriel, J. D. and Ridgway, G. L. (1989). *Chlamydia trachomatis* infection in a gynaecology clinic population: identification of high-risk groups and the value of contact tracing. *Euro. J. Obstet. Gyn. Reprod. Biol.*, **31**, 67–74.

10. Templeton, A. (Ed.) (1996). *The Prevention of Pelvic Infection*, RCOG Press, 267.

10 – Workgroup 3: Improving Access to Sexual Health Services, and Sexual Health Promotion

Group Facilitators: *Toni Belfield and Anne Scoular*

Group Rapporteur: *Toni Belfield*

Workgroup 3 consisted of professionals working in the fields of family planning, genitourinary medicine, obstetrics and gynaecology, research and health promotion.

Improving Access to Sexual Health Services

In any discussion looking at improving access to sexual health services, there has to be a common agreement on how sexual health is defined. The 'Greenhouse' definition discussed during the Consensus Workshop (Appendix 1) was agreed, and is:

> *'Sexual health is the enjoyment of sexual activity of one's choice, without causing or suffering physical or mental harm.'*

The proposal to adopt the Greenhouse definition recognised the need for a concise definition of sexual health which unites both benefits and deficits. Greenhouse indicates that any definition should be simple, understandable, memorable, applicable to a wide range of social, religious and sexual cultures, robust enough to stand critical analysis and sufficiently unambiguous as to be capable of expansion without significant distortion.

Sexual health services naturally encompass family planning (FP) and sexually transmitted diseases (STDs). Both areas are characterised by intrinsic similarities and fundamental differences. Both have been identified by policy makers as important public health priorities (*The Health of the Nation*, 1992). As such, strategies to improve collaboration between the different sexual health disciplines are being welcomed by all in the field in order to provide more considered and consistent approaches to sexual health promotion and provision.

The term 'sexual health services' is a relatively new concept; for many, it only relates to FP and genitourinary medicine (GUM). However, to be effective for the future, collaborative approaches to sexual health *must* recognise and respect the expertise of *all* the different contributing disciplines.

Currently, existing sexual health services are provided through a variety of outlets and in a number of different ways. These may not always be known to purchasers, providers, or, importantly, to service users (actual or potential). The goal of any service is to attract and be accessible to clients who need or wish to use it. At the time of writing there is little national information on sexual health services, for example:

- Who uses services or do not use services.
- Why services are used or not used.
- How services are accessed.
- Where services are.
- Whether services are liked, disliked or meet actual or perceived needs.

The motivation to use FP services or GUM services can be viewed as very different:

- FP services are used primarily to prevent or plan something happening in the future (pregnancy).
- GUM services are available to sort out something that has already happened (infection).

- Professionals and users see the different services as having restricted roles with discrete populations.
- Communication to date between the two disciplines has been limited, which has resulted in a lack of standardised procedures and guidelines addressing service delivery, treatments and referral.

In order to improve 'accessibility' to sexual health services (defined in the *Oxford Dictionary* as 'opportunity of getting there') there needs to be an understanding of the general barriers that surround FP (contraception) *and* STDs.

Existing barriers to using FP and GUM services do have some commonality which can be divided into 'service barriers' (access, promotion, availability) and 'people barriers' (embarrassment, discomfort, knowledge).

Service Barriers

- What services offer.
- Where to find information about services (for example, there are no standardised listings in telephone directors for FP clinics or GUM services).
- Non-generic names are given to services (e.g. Margaret Pyke Centre, Martha and Luke Clinics, Clinic 11, Mortimer Market).
- It can be very difficult trying to locate an FP clinic, and far worse trying to access information about a GUM service.
- Locality of services – towns and rural, various problems of transport to reach the services.
- Location of clinics – some GUM services are still located in the bowels of the hospital.
- Times of opening.
- Appointment systems or open access non-appointment sessions.
- Waiting times.
- Staffing of clinics (male/female staff, clinical/non-clinical).
- Attitudes of staff working in clinics.
- Lack of accessible, impartial and up-to-date written information.

People Barriers

- Age.
- Ethnicity.
- Sex, gender and sexual orientation.
- Social and cultural background.
- Aspects of disability.
- Historical and current aspects of stigmatisation of services and users.

To improve access, the Working Group provided the following recommendations:

- Recognise and address the barriers to access which relate to the professionals' roles, service delivery, clinic services and information giving.
- Prioritise the standardisation of listings for FP and GUM services in local telephone directories throughout the UK.
- Shift the focus of sexual health services to promote the idea of sexual health, rather than illness or risk, making it positive rather than negative.
- Recognise the need to maintain the flexibility of sexual health services through a variety of outlets – this is a major strength, *not* a weakness.
- Address the need for better standardisation of procedures through agreed guidelines and protocols for audit. The aim is to improve service delivery, treatments and information giving.
- Undertake needs assessment at a local level to plan the provision of equally accessible services.
- Services should work towards incorporating sessions for people with specific needs, in order to demonstrate that services welcome these groups and are sensitive to their needs.
- Collect and co-ordinate the projects and research UK wide to prevent reinventing the wheel.
- Recognise that sexual health services cannot always be all things to all people.
- Address issues of stigma.

Sexual Health Promotion

Sexual health promotion is a broad concept that involves activities that *promote* informed choices in relation to sexual health.

The area of sexual health is a multidisciplinary one; indeed, this is its strength. It is vital to recognise that issues of sexual health cross *all* areas of health and cannot be neatly packaged or compartmentalised. As such there is a need to develop future strategies that allow for:

- The development of a district-wide sexual health strategy which encompasses clinical, medical and educational areas, and recognises and supports outlets in a variety of settings.
- Recognise that within any sexual health strategy there is a need for 'horizontal' and 'vertical' integration between providers and within provider units.
- The development of mechanisms in each area where GUM professionals and FP professionals know about and visit each other's services.
- Support for professionals working in sexual health services who need to be proactive in promoting their services and being positive about what they have to offer.
- Improved knowledge and studies in the area of sexual health promotion which need to be brought together through some form of clearing house to maximise knowledge and resources and to prevent duplication of effort.
- Provision of effective monitoring activities which are required in the area of sexual health promotion.
- Support, development and recognition of the pivotal role that health promotion services can and do play in developing and supporting sexual health promotion in a wide range of medical and non-medical settings.
- Support and development of the role of education at primary, secondary and higher education levels.
- Recognition and effective use of the media in promoting the positive and beneficial aspects of sexual health.
- Recognition for the need for effective communication skills in all areas of sexual health promotion and sexual health delivery.

11 – Workgroup 4: Training, Evaluation and Research

Derek Timmins

Group Facilitator: *Meera Kishen*

Group Rapporteur: *Derek Temmins*

Introduction

In the UK, genitourinary medicine (GUM) and family planning services (FPS) provide for different patient needs but with an important degree of overlap in these services. Traditionally, GUM has always been a hospital-laboratory-based service while FP occupies locations in the community (20%) and general practice (80%).

The importance of sexual health was indicated by its inclusion as one of the key service area objectives in *The Health of the Nation* and the extensive use of services (GUM/FP) made by patients. The service structure provides for excellence with its concentration of specialist expertise. In GUM and FP, Korner data collection and analysis generate important epidemiological data. Co-ordinated teaching/research and audit is well established in GUM and in many (but not all) FP clinics.

If we are to further improve sexual health in the UK, it will be important to build on the success (agreement will be needed on suitable measures of success) of these services and to foster closer relevant links and alliances which will benefit patient care and better meet patient needs. These might take the form of loose linkage or formal structural changes to integrate services. The format will be dictated by local context and needs, etc.

Central to improvements in the future will be an enhanced integrated teaching/training and research/audit programme so as to foster closer collaboration and partnership in care with the aim of better meeting patients' needs, better shared understandings, better health promotion, and improved prevention and control strategies. The last mentioned is particularly relevant, for example, between GUM and FP. Ultimately this implies a degree of cultural shift and closer working, and a synergic relationship between GUM and FP services, while at the same time maintaining the generic identity of each service.

Particularly important is the need to ensure that this hub of cutting edge expertise continues to inform and influence related care in general practice. A successful integrated training formula can form a recipe for better integration of services.

Training Needs

The implementation of Calman has meant that detailed curricula for higher specialist training now exist for GUM but not yet for FP/reproductive healthcare. The latter are being developed.

Identified subject areas requiring training can be divided as follows:

1. Detailed clinical knowledge and skills in the following subjects:
   (a) Sexually transmitted diseases including HIV/AIDS and palliative care.
   (b) Contraception/reproductive health. To include termination of pregnancy.
   (c) Psychosexual medicine/marital therapy.
   (d) Colposcopy.
   (e) Sexual assault/abuse.
   (f) Menopause and hormone replacement therapy.
2. Communication and inter-personal skills. Training would include media skill and internal/ external PR issues.

3. Research, clinical audit, quality management, computer and information management skills.
4. Educational/teaching skills/training the trainers.
5. Interface with obstetrics and gynaecology (women's health care) and primary care – this would include general practitioners, other community providers, practice nurses, and voluntary services/women's health and sexual health information services.
6. Management skills – to include concepts of leadership, creative management, time management/organisation skills, teams, marketing and image management, the internal and external environments.
7. Screening issues related to cytology and genital tract infections.

Current Training Programmes

Having identified the core elements of a desirable shared curriculum, the scrutiny of current training in GUM and FP reveals a lack of integration, gaps and overlap. The existing individual training programme of each speciality alone does not address all the relevant issues which make a comprehensive integrated sexual health service.

If the concept of an integrated sexual health service is to be applied, then a new integrated curriculum combining the training areas identified above would need to be agreed. To meet the needs of modern times, this would be modular so as to be flexible and offer choice in relation to the training needs of specific groups of service providers.

Recommendations

To form a joint educational group to agree the core and peripheral curricula in detail. This would include inputs from GUM/FP/ GP/nursing and other relevant groups.

Key target groups for training would include:

1. Doctors

- Undergraduates
- GUM (postgraduate/career)
- General practitioners
- FP (postgraduate/career)
- Obstetricians and gynaecologists
- Nursing staff
- Current training programmes, including Dip GUM, MSc GUM, MRCGP, DFFP and MFFP.

2. Nurses

- General practice
- Schools
- Family planning
- Genitourinary medicine
- Others

Current training includes ENB 934, ENB 901, ENB 908, Marie Curie Centre.

3. Administrative and key support workers

- Health advisers
- Counsellors
- General practice link workers
- Social workers
- Receptionists

4. Other providers working with individuals and groups with un-met sexual health needs and awareness of services available

- Outreach workers
- The homeless
- Women's health information groups
- Men's health groups
- Peer educators
- Young persons' groups
- Universities and colleges

- Others to be identified
- Charitable groups, e.g. Brook

In moving to set up a new integrated training opportunity in sexual health, the following elements would be particularly desirable:

1. Co-ordinated sharing of staff across general practice/hospital and family planning settings. More use of exchange staff and secondments, ideally with placements being at least for one month at a time.
2. To set up a directory of existing training facilities and review content, coverage and relevance in relation to identifying potential resources for teaching an integrated sexual health curriculum.
3. To continue to identify training needs aligned to patient needs through the process of clinical audit.
4. FP clinics and general practice to develop shared care guidelines and to continually refine the same.
5. An integrated training programme will include theoretical and experiential/skills teaching elements.
6. There is a need for a steering committee to address in detail the current gaps, training needs and structure for a sexual health curriculum and to construct a core and peripheral curriculum presented in modular form offering choice in the range and level of training achieved. It is envisaged that training would be theoretical, practical with skill and inter-personal emphasis, group and problem based, experiential, role play, discussion groups, project based, etc. The availability of a modular format would allow for flexibility and for staff to acquire additional skills aligned to their changing workplace needs.

Emphasis should be placed on achieving the right balance of knowledge, skills and attitudes so as to deliver an optimal package of care at the minimum possible cost.

If adopted, such an integrated curriculum concept would involve much work and a division of labour with experts being given the remit to address specific areas and with suitable control processes to co-ordinate the exercise. Agreed documents would then be reviewed and refined by an interactive process of consultation within the faculty and validated by appropriate reference groups. If adopted, the exercise would require a level of resourcing yet to be identified.

Having generated the concept of an integrated sexual health training curriculum, the group then addressed the issue of research and evaluation of services related to sexual health. The objectives chosen included:

1. To ascertain why patients access services and the reasons for the current patterns of use.
2. To identify users' sexual health needs and to identify what needs are not currently met by existing services and the hierarchy of priority of these health needs.
3. To investigate users' perceptions of service/care priorities.
4. To investigate GP perceptions of service/care priorities and preferred models of sexual health service delivery with reasons and explanations.
5. Research on determinants of risk-taking behaviours and success or otherwise of intervention aimed at achieving behavioural change conducive to better sexual health.
6. Sexual health – patient issues:
   - Need for reassurance and anxiety reduction.
   - Doctor/patient communication issues.
   - Psychosexual issues.
   - Education of patients in negotiation skills, role play, social scripting, etc.
   - Need for advice about STDs and other genital concerns including body image/self esteem and personal constructs.
   - Education on sexual/relational matters to enhance quality of life relationships and personal understanding.
7. To investigate patient knowledge, desires, preferences, wants and expectations of services.
8. To assess current provision and current patient needs and identify service gaps.
9. To assess the effectiveness of health promotion and behavioural intervention strategies.

Subjects for Research

Genitourinary Medicine

1. STD incidence prevalence and cure rates.
2. Sexual behaviour – to identify changes in behaviour. We need to define a core set of behaviours, related questions and provide a risk score.
3. Partner notification effectiveness.
4. To investigate the availability, accuracy, timeliness, relevance and consistency of health information and messages provided to patients.
5. Unmet patient needs, e.g. commercial sex workers.
6. Ethnic minority groups and STDs.
7. Incidence and range of presenting psychosexual complaints.
8. Patient satisfaction surveys.
9. Piloting and use of national audit instruments for gonorrhoea, partner notification, *Chlamydia* and genital herpes management.
10. To establish a model for the extended role of the nurse in GUM/FP clinics.
11. To investigate patient preference and choice in place of treatment of STDs.
12. To evaluate the content and effectiveness of sexual health education in GUM.

Family Planning

1. To investigate cost-effectiveness of FP services.
2. User perceptions of FP services in comparison to user perceptions of GP services for FP.
3. Research on range, uptake and costs of existing services. A more co-ordinated collection and dissemination of such data.
4. To pilot and evaluate outcomes of different models of GUM/FP clinics/GP collaborative care.
5. To identify consumer priorities and the hierarchy of priority determining their choice for using particular services.
6. To research and improve existing FP clinical provisions.

7. To evaluate the content and effectiveness of sexual health education in the FP setting.
8. To investigate young persons' use of non-GP- and GP-based FP services.

Appendix 1 Consensus Workshop on Sexually Transmitted Diseases and Contraception: Sexual Health Promotion and Service Delivery

The Steering Group: Caroline Bradbeer, Ali Kubba, Jayshree Pillaye, Sarah Randall and Helen Ward

The Consensus Statement

We define sexual health as the enjoyment of sexual activity of one's choice, without causing or suffering physical or mental harm. The components of sexual health services include the prevention and management of sexually transmitted diseases (STDs) and unintended pregnancies, the prevention of reproductive morbidity and the management of sexual dysfunction.

There are many people and agencies involved in the promotion of sexual health and the provision of related health services. There are three major providers of specific sexual health services within the NHS – the primary health care team, family planning clinics and departments of genitourinary medicine. In addition, education services, social services, the voluntary sector, various community organisations and the health service in general have a role to play in the promotion of sexual health.

Family planning and genitourinary medicine services are open access permitting self-referral, and are provided free of charge in

97

the interests of public health. Each provides one or more elements of a sexual health service, but neither speciality covers all aspects.

In order to maximise health gain in this area, and in particular to meet the objectives outlined in strategy documents such as *The Health of the Nation*, we recommend the following objectives as the bases of a strategy for sexual health services:

- To protect and strengthen the public health by maintaining the provision of free sexual health services to which people can refer themselves, and which are appropriate to local needs.
- To move towards greater convergence of the various sexual health services in order to ensure that people using the services have access to an appropriate range of care at one time, in response to expressed wishes.
- To utilise such convergence to reduce multiple attendances and maximise the effective use of resources.

Appropriate models of care will differ according to the setting, ranging from collaboration between specialist services (genito-urinary medicine, family planning, health promotion), to a fully integrated sexual health service providing a full range of health promotion and care facilities.

To ensure that we make progress towards these objectives, in-tegrated strategies are needed at a local and national level. Public health specialists can play a leading role by promoting an integra-ted purchasing strategy through working with GP fundholders and commissioning agencies. An integrated strategy should aim to protect open access services for the whole population, through core funding for genitourinary medicine and family planning services.

The initial step in this direction is the setting up of a local strategy forum, involving providers, public health specialists, general practitioners and commissioners. These groups should consider the range of services available locally and the develop-ment of high quality specialist sexual health services through a greater convergence of family planning and genitourinary medicine. Purchasers should consider the way in which primary care interfaces with, and receives support from, these specialised services. Such a forum could also play a key role in ensuring an integrated health promotion and sex education strategy, making maximum use of all opportunities for promoting sexual health.

We therefore need:

- To retain patient choice in the provision of sexual health services.
- Adequate funding to ensure that these services remain free and open access.
- Shared guidelines across the sectors (family planning, genito-urinary medicine, general practice), outlining good practice and agreed minimum standards and facilities.
- Properly funded and supported training to implement these guidelines; this could include the exchange of staff to promote the sharing of skills.
- To ensure that services address the diversity of need in their community.
- Evaluation and monitoring of services, to include user perspective and cost-effectiveness.
- Co-ordination of health promotion activities to make best use of opportunities for sex education and health promotion within the services and in the community.
- Research to underpin guidelines for good clinical practice, effective health promotion and appropriate service provision.

Appendix 2 The Participants and their Affiliations

Dr Sheila Adams, Director of Public Health, North Thames Health
Authority

Ms Isobel Allen, Policy Studies Institute

Dr Anura Alawattegama, Consultant Physician, Department of
Genitourinary Medicine, Royal Liverpool University Hospital

Mr Peter Bellamy, Commissioner for Sexual Health, HIV Services
Department, Edgbaston

Ms Toni Belfield, Head of Information and Research, FPA

Dr Anona Blackwell, Consultant in GUM, Singleton Hospital

Ms Rochelle Bloch, Senior Commissioning Manager – HIV and
AIDS, Ealing, Hammersmith and Hounslow Health Agency

Dr Caroline Bradbeer, Consultant Physician, Lydia Department of
Genitourinary Medicine, St Thomas' Hospital

Mr David R. Bronham, Senior Lecturer and Chairman FFP &
RHC

Ms Gillian Butler, London

Dr Penny Chandiok, Consultant Physician, Department of
Genitourinary Medicine, Withington Hospital, Manchester

Dr Elaine Cooper, Senior Clinical Medical Officer, Central Clinic,
Southampton

Dr Eric Curless, Consultant Physician, Department of
Genitourinary Medicine, Bolton General Hospital

Dr Stephen Dawson, Consultant Physician, Genitourinary
Medicine, Garden Clinic, Upton Hospital

Mr David Evans, Research Fellow, Institute of Health Policy

Study

Ms Clare Farquhar, Honorary Researcher, Health Promotion Services, St Pancras Hospital

Dr Mark Fitzgerald, Consultant in Genitourinary Medicine and President MSSVD, Somerset and Taunton Hospital

Mr Peter Greenhouse, Consultant in Sexual Health, Department of Sexual Health

Dr Mary Hepburn, Senior Lecturer – Obstetrics and Gynaecology, Glasgow Royal Maternity Hospital

Mrs Muriel Holroyd, Chair Elect, RCN Family Planning Forum

Dr Jennifer Hopwood, Senior Clinical Medical Officer in Family Planning, The Wirral

Dr Anne Johnson, Reader, Academic Department of Genitourinary Medicine, Mortimer Market Centre, London

Dr Rosemary Kirkman, Consultant in Family Planning and Reproductive Health, Department of Obstetrics and Gynaecology, University of Manchester

Dr Meera Kishen, Consultant in Family Planning and Reproductive Health, Liverpool

Dr Ali Kubba, Consultant Community Gynaecologist, West Lambeth Family Planning and Reproductive Health Service

Dr Paul Loo, Consultant in Genitourinary Medicine, Kettering General Hospital

Ms Wendy Majewska, Vice President SHASTD, Department of Genitourinary Medicine, St George's Hospital

Dr Helen Massil, Consultant in Family Planning and Reproductive Health, Optimum – St Giles

Dr Colin Mathews, General Practitioner, Portadown

Dr Patrick Morgan, Consultant in Communicable Disease Control, Northamptonshire Health Authority

Dr Helen McGuire, Regional Epidemiologist, South Thames RHA

Dr John Modle, Department of Health

Ms Mary Packer

Dr Stephen Peckham, Institute of Health Policy Studies, Faculty of Social Sciences, University of Southampton

Dr Jayshree Pillaye, Senior Doctor, Health Education Authority, London

Dr Sarah Randall, Consultant in Family Planning and Reproductive Health, Portsmouth

Dr Roland Salmon, Chairman, Working Group on Sexual Health and HIV Infection – FPHM, Consultant Epidemiologist, PHLS CDSC (Welsh Unit), Cardiff

Dr Anne Scoular, Consultant in Genitourinary Medicine, Glasgow Royal Infirmary

Dr Connie Smith, Director, Women's Services, Parkside Health

Dr Alfie Sparks, Consultant in Genitourinary Medicine, Cardiff Royal Infirmary

Dr Lindy Stacey, Consultant Community Gynaecologist, City and Hackney Health Trust

Dr Yvonne Stedman, Consultant in Family Planning and Reproductive Health Care, Worcester

Dr Alison Stirland, Clinical Medical Officer in Family Planning, City and Hackney Trust

Ms Sue Sullivan, Community Nurse Manager, South Kent NHS Community Trust

Dr Nicol Thin, Consultant Physician, Lydia Department of Genitourinary Medicine, St Thomas' Hospital

Dr Derek Timmins, Consultant Physician, Department of Genitourinary Medicine, Royal Liverpool University Hospital

Ms Pat Tweed, Staffordshire

Dr Helen Ward, Senior Lecturer in Public Health, St Mary's Hospital Medical School, London

Dr Sarah Wilson, Senior Lecturer in Public Health Medicine, Medical School, Queen's Medical Centre

Dr Jennifer Wordsworth, Family Planning and Women's Health, Sheffield

Dr Richard Wrigley, General Practitioner, London

Appendix 3   Acknowledgements

The Steering Group is most grateful for the generous support of the Consensus Workshops from the following:

Health Education Authority
North Thames Regional Health Authority
South Thames Regional Health Authority
Janssen-Cilag
Organon Laboratories
Schering Healthcare
Sutherland Health
Wyeth Laboratories

The following also sponsored this publication:

Janssen-Cilag
Organon Laboratories
Schering Healthcare
Sutherland Health